STATISTICAL EXERCIS[...]
MEDICAL RESEARCH

TO THE STUDENTS

IT HAS BEEN MY PRIVILEGE

TO TEACH

STATISTICAL EXERCISES IN MEDICAL RESEARCH

JOHN F. OSBORN

BSc, PhD

Lecturer in Medical Demography,
London School of Hygiene and
Tropical Medicine
University of London

FOREWORD BY
P. ARMITAGE
Professor of Biomathematics
University of Oxford

BLACKWELL SCIENTIFIC PUBLICATIONS

OXFORD LONDON EDINBURGH MELBOURNE

© 1979 Blackwell Scientific Publications
Osney Mead, Oxford ox2 0EL
8 John Street, London, wc1n 2es
9 Forrest Road, Edinburgh, eh1 2qh
P.O. Box 9, North Balwyn, Victoria 3104, Australia

First published 1979

British Library Cataloguing in Publication Data

Osborn, John F
    Statistical exercises in medical research.
    1. Mathematical statistics
    2. Medical statistics
    I. Title
    519.5′02′461   QA276

    ISBN 0–632–00026–0

Distributed in North America by
Halsted Press, a division of
John Wiley & Sons Inc.
605 Third Avenue, New York, NY 10016

Printed in Great Britain by
Western Printing Services Ltd,
Avonmouth
and bound by
Kemp Hall Bindery
Oxford

CONTENTS*

* Chapter and section numbers and titles correspond to those in Armitage P. (1971) *Statistical Methods in Medical Research*, Blackwell Scientific Publications, Oxford.

FOREWORD

Statistical methods are the techniques which have been developed for the collection, processing and interpretation of real data. Any course in statistics which avoids substantial contact with data therefore presents a very restrictive view of the subject. By studying a variety of data sets the student, whether a future statistician or a scientific research worker, is able to grasp the context in which particular methods are appropriate and to become more fluent in the use of these methods.

Textbooks on mathematical statistics usually include theoretical exercises. Those on applied statistics are less likely to include comparable practical exercises because of the space required and the task of finding sensible data. Dr Osborn has performed a valuable service in compiling the present collection. The data are taken predominantly from medical research projects, and the techniques which the reader is invited to apply cover a wide spectrum of commonly-used methods. The collection will be of great value as an adjunct to courses on medical and biological statistics, and for all those who wish to obtain more experience in the practical use of statistical methods.

P. ARMITAGE
Professor of Biomathematics
University of Oxford

PREFACE

Teaching medical statistics to post-graduate medical students during the past decade or so, has taught me that lectures, seminars and textbooks are not sufficient to ensure that the statistical material intended to be taught, is in fact learned. At the London School of Hygiene and Tropical Medicine, each one hour lecture in medical statistics is followed by practical work lasting about one and a half hours. Despite this, it is very common for students to request further exercises to ensure that the learning objectives of the lecture are in fact realized. Thus this book of exercises is intended to help students and medical research workers who, having received instruction in the methods of medical statistics, wish to confirm their ability to apply the techniques to data. The students at the London School of Hygiene and Tropical Medicine have interests in a wide variety of medical specialities including, for example, community medicine, medical demography, epidemiology, human nutrition, occupational health, tropical medicine and so on. The exercises in this book have been selected from a similarly wide variety of subjects in order to provide a balance which, it is hoped will be of interest to all medical research workers, whatever their speciality.

Since its publication, *Statistical Methods in Medical Research* (Armitage P. (1971) Blackwell Scientific Publications, Oxford), has established itself as a standard text and reference work among both students and research workers in medicine and *Statistical Exercises in Medical Research* is intended to be a companion volume, the chapter and section titles being common to both books for ease of reference. This, however, has led to some anomalies in the numbering of some sections in *Statistical Exercises in Medical Research*. For example, Chapter 1 starts at section 1.2, since in *Statistical Methods in Medical Research* section 1.1 is devoted to a general discussion of the application of statistical methods to medical problems, for which it is difficult to envisage appropriate statistical exercises for the reader. Section 1.2 in both books is headed Diagrams.

JOHN F. OSBORN

ACKNOWLEDGEMENTS

In any book such as this, which is to a large extent, the result of the author's teaching experience, any complete list of acknowledgements would be excessively long. I am very grateful to all my colleagues, friends and students who have made contributions to this book. However, several people have given very specific help and, in particular, I must thank Professor Peter Armitage who first suggested to me that a book of statistical exercises would be useful to medical students and medical research workers, and who has helped and encouraged me throughout its preparation. Some of the exercises have been used at the London School of Hygiene and Tropical Medicine in the courses of medical statistics for many years, and I am grateful to Professor Armitage, Professor William Brass, Dr Paul Fine, Dr Ronald H. Gray and other colleagues who originally abstracted this data from the literature. For assistance with the checking of answers and advice on computing I thank Miss Patricia E. Doyle and Ms Basia Zaba. The typescript was read by Professor Armitage, Professor Brass, Professor Michael R.H. Healy, my wife, Mrs Erica M. Osborn and my father Mr Frederick J. Osborn, all of whom made suggestions which improved the exercises.

I am also grateful to Miss Sandra A. Etheridge whose expertise has enabled the manuscript to be typed quickly and accurately. Miss Dorothy E. Boyes and Miss Sue M. Evans gave additional secretarial help.

Finally, I must thank all those workers in medical research whose efforts have produced the data for these exercises. References to the origin of data have been given where these have been traced, but some of the material, particularly data which have been tailored for use as teaching material in the London School of Hygiene and Tropical Medicine for many years, is given without reference.

If, despite the valuable assistance I have received, there are residual errors, these are entirely my responsibility, and I would be grateful to have them pointed out to me.

JOHN F. OSBORN

CHAPTER 1

THE SCOPE OF STATISTICS

1.2 DIAGRAMS

1.2.1 The data below show the numbers of neonatal and post-neonatal deaths recorded during each month of 1951 in England and Wales. (A neonatal death is the death of an infant within 28 days of birth; a post-neonatal death is the death of an infant aged between 29 days and one year.) Calculate the average number of neonatal and post-neonatal deaths per day, for each month and plot these to indicate the differences in seasonal trend.

Month	Neonatal deaths	Post-neonatal deaths
January	1224	1080
February	1099	872
March	1271	923
April	1141	705
May	1137	553
June	1077	410
July	959	408
August	952	381
September	907	390
October	982	444
November	973	493
December	1036	699
Total	12,758	7358

1.2.2 The crude birth rate (CBR) and the crude death rate (CDR) for England and Wales from 1926 are shown below. The difference between these two rates is called the crude rate of natural increase (CRNI). Plot graphs of these three rates to show their trends since 1926.

Rates per 1,000 population				Rates per 1,000 population			
Year	CBR	CDR	CRNI	Year	CBR	CDR	CRNI
1926	17·8	11·6	6·2	1952	15·3	11·3	4·0
1927	16·7	12·3	4·4	1953	15·5	11·4	4·1
1928	16·7	11·7	5·0	1954	15·2	11·3	3·9
1929	16·3	13·4	2·9	1955	15·0	11·7	3·3
1930	16·3	11·4	4·9	1956	15·7	11·7	4·0
1931	15·8	12·3	3·5	1957	16·1	11·5	4·6
1932	15·3	12·0	3·3	1958	16·4	11·7	4·7
1933	14·4	12·3	2·1	1959	16·5	11·6	4·9
1934	14·8	11·8	3·0	1960	17·1	11·5	5·6
1935	14·7	11·7	3·0	1961	17·6	11·9	5·7
1936	14·8	12·1	2·7	1962	18·0	11·9	6·1
1937	14·9	12·4	2·5	1963	18·2	12·2	6·0
1938	15·1	11·6	3·5	1964	18·6	11·3	7·3
1939	14·8	12·1	2·7	1965	18·1	11·5	6·6
1940	14·1	14·4	−0·3	1966	17·8	11·7	6·1
1941	13·9	13·5	0·4	1967	17·3	11·2	6·1
1942	15·6	12·3	3·3	1968	16·9	11·9	5·0
1943	16·2	13·0	3·2	1969	16·4	11·9	4·5
1944	17·7	12·7	5·0	1970	16·1	11·7	4·4
1945	15·9	12·6	3·3	1971	16·0	11·6	4·4
1946	19·2	12·0	7·2	1972	14·8	12·0	2·8
1947	20·5	12·3	8·2	1973	13·7	11·8	1·9
1948	17·8	11·0	6·8	1974	13·0	11·8	1·2
1949	16·7	11·8	4·9	1975	12·2	11·7	0·5
1950	15·8	11·6	4·2	1976	11·9	12·0	−0·1
1951	15·5	12·5	3·0				

1.2.3 The data below show the percentage of the population of England and Wales who are of pensionable age (i.e. males aged 65+ and females 60+ years of age).

(a) Draw a graph to illustrate the trend in the percentage of persons of pensionable age during the period 1901–1971.

(b) How might this trend affect the trend in the crude death rate during this period? (See for example exercise 1.2.2.)

Year	1901	1911	1921	1931	1941	1951	1961	1971
%	6·2	6·8	7.9	9·6	11·8	13·6	14·6	16·0

1.4 SUMMARIZING NUMERICAL DATA

1.4.1 The recorded birth weights of 18,645 singleton live and stillbirths occurring in South-West England in 1965 are given below. There is some evidence of digit preference particularly at zero and 8 ounce points. Using one pound weight intervals construct a frequency distribution and a relative frequency distribution. Draw a histogram to illustrate the data.

Distribution of Recorded Birth Weight, South-West of England, 1965
Number of Singleton, Live and Stillbirths

Pounds	Ounces															
	0	1	2	3	4	5	6	7	8	9	10	11	12	13	14	15
0	0	0	0	0	0	0	0	0	0	0	0	0	1	0	0	2
1	6	1	1	1	3	0	2	2	3	1	3	4	8	2	2	1
2	18	4	2	2	6	2	4	2	10	4	4	2	8	7	4	3
3	14	6	8	5	9	6	8	9	14	2	6	6	7	5	14	7
4	22	14	16	19	16	14	15	19	47	17	23	15	39	30	26	32
5	66	37	42	46	60	41	67	59	106	78	98	68	135	92	106	81
6	323	101	183	157	337	160	205	172	504	215	299	222	496	256	315	228
7	914	225	390	286	697	311	417	291	817	289	369	279	626	246	330	236
8	920	195	292	220	508	200	230	166	485	147	198	110	288	122	146	78
9	395	83	118	72	142	53	69	45	145	35	42	22	91	18	25	10
10	88	12	26	9	23	11	6	4	18	8	7	2	16	4	2	4
11	17	1	3	2	3	1	0	2	2	0	4	1	2	0	1	0
12	2	0	0	0	0	0	0	0	0	0	0	0	0	0	0	0
13	0	0	0	0	0	0	0	0	0	0	0	0	0	0	0	0
14	1	0	0	0	0	0	0	0	0	0	0	0	0	0	0	0

Total, including 51 with unknown birth weight: 18,696

Source: Pethybridge R.J., Ashford J.R. & Fryer J.G. (1974) *Brit. J. prev. soc. Med.* **28**, 10–18.

1.4.2 The distributions in the first table below show the pre-operational percentage haemoglobin values of a sample of the population of a village where there has been a malaria eradication programme (MEP).

The results in a sample obtained after MEP are given in the second table.

Construct similar distributions for these post-operational percentage haemoglobin values. Compare the relative frequency distribution observed before MEP with that obtained after MEP.

Haemoglobin %	30–39	40–49	50–59	60–69	70–79	80–89	90–99	100–109	Total
Frequency	2	7	14	10	8	2	2	0	45
% of total	4·4	15·6	31·1	22·2	17·8	4·4	4·4	0	99·9

43	63	63	75	95	75	80	48	62	71	76	90
51	61	74	103	93	82	74	65	63	53	64	67
80	77	60	69	73	76	91	55	65	69	84	78
50	68	72	89	75	57	66	79	85	70	59	71
87	67	72	52	35	67	99	81	97	74	61	72

1.4.3 Detailed studies on filariasis in Fiji required that a census be made of the population. Data for 8 villages on the islands of Taveuni and Koro are given below. (*Report to the Director of Medical Services, Fiji*, 1968–1969.)

Draw a histogram to show the percentage distribution of the population of males by age.

Draw a cumulative relative frequency distribution. From the graph of the cumulative distribution determine the age which divides the population 50–50, i.e. at what age, say x years, are 50% of the males younger than x and 50% older than x?

Age last birthday	No. males	% of total males
0–4	154	18·6
5–9	135	16·3
10–14	107	12·9
15–19	72	8·7
20–29	112	13·5
30–39	97	11·7
40–49	67	8·1
50–59	47	5·7
60–79	39	4·7
Total	830	100·2

1.4.4 Using 2 mm grouping intervals, construct a frequency distribution and relative frequency distribution of the skinfold thicknesses given in the table below. The measurements given are skinfold thicknesses in millimetres at the triceps mid-point for 121 male subjects.

11·4	15·3	9·1	18·4	10·9	4·7	9·6	20·6	10·4	20·5	22·4
14·3	11·7	11·4	12·7	18·2	15·1	14·6	25·3	11·5	13·2	7·9
12·6	13·9	16·8	11·4	27·3	16·3	13·9	13·2	11·9	20·0	13·2
9·4	18·9	10·7	14·8	17·8	10·8	16·0	15·7	17·7	13·5	11·5
11·1	9·6	15·1	13·6	13·6	8·6	6·9	19·1	18·7	10·1	16·0
20·4	7·9	16·6	18·5	16·2	17·4	18·8	12·6	22·0	9·6	11·1
15·7	23·7	13·3	4·9	8·3	20·1	15·5	23·1	10·2	10·7	15·8
17·6	21·3	16·2	14·9	9·9	9·1	9·9	9·8	8·6	11·8	9·3
14·8	17·3	9·5	13·6	12·4	9·5	14·3	25·7	12·9	22·7	12·1
10·7	16·8	11·3	11·3	11·4	5·9	10·7	14·6	19·8	25·5	7·7
18·4	7·9	7·6	23·3	9·6	8·4	10·4	8·1	12·5	9·0	30·1

Source: Colley J.R.T., personal communication; *see also* Ruiz L., Colley J.R.T. & Hamilton P.J.S. (1971) *Brit. J. prev. soc. Med.* **25**, 165–167.

B

THE SCOPE OF STATISTICS

1.4.5 The sprayable surface area (in square feet) of the 250 houses of an African village are shown below. Using class widths of 10 square feet construct a frequency distribution of the sprayable surface areas.

No.	Area	No.	Area	No.	Area	No.	Area	No.	Area	No.	Area	No.	Area
1	216	41	328	81	185	121	236	161	254	201	286	241	173
2	231	42	262	82	233	122	219	162	238	202	192	242	208
3	194	43	282	83	214	123	255	163	274	203	300	243	283
4	188	44	221	84	237	124	245	164	265	204	276	244	253
5	326	45	243	85	271	125	257	165	234	205	291	245	227
6	214	46	241	86	263	126	191	166	224	206	191	246	242
7	264	47	203	87	261	127	284	167	212	207	291	247	231
8	255	48	168	88	307	128	211	168	249	208	290	248	250
9	242	49	258	89	215	129	293	169	254	209	211	249	229
10	305	50	234	90	261	130	184	170	234	210	280	250	287
11	311	51	314	91	256	131	219	171	217	211	258		
12	300	52	259	92	224	132	272	172	247	212	200		
13	254	53	301	93	259	133	251	173	206	213	234		
14	193	54	219	94	221	134	272	174	283	214	263		
15	245	55	282	95	239	135	254	175	264	215	236		
16	165	56	303	96	230	136	271	176	332	216	245		
17	201	57	207	97	257	137	222	177	219	217	254		
18	241	58	283	98	237	138	266	178	262	218	249		
19	220	59	204	99	238	139	281	179	319	219	258		
20	240	60	264	100	257	140	227	180	338	220	207		
21	281	61	281	101	296	141	259	181	309	221	225		
22	261	62	270	102	266	142	235	182	318	222	252		
23	320	63	196	103	285	143	223	183	327	223	281		
24	240	64	204	104	315	144	243	184	298	224	253		
25	259	65	233	105	237	145	255	185	196	225	210		
26	292	66	239	106	234	146	268	186	262	226	228		
27	184	67	255	107	181	147	282	187	242	227	230		
28	320	68	325	108	193	148	253	188	261	228	261		
29	269	69	289	109	256	149	226	189	258	229	194		
30	277	70	263	110	247	150	248	190	305	230	304		
31	285	71	251	111	269	151	303	191	285	231	227		
32	318	72	246	112	218	152	301	192	256	232	243		
33	258	73	222	113	329	153	254	193	228	233	271		
34	182	74	205	114	227	154	244	194	209	234	326		
35	199	75	170	115	284	155	228	195	244	235	278		
36	294	76	209	116	255	156	271	196	251	236	272		
37	286	77	310	117	250	157	269	197	232	237	267		
38	203	78	272	118	269	158	316	198	171	238	285		
39	266	79	288	119	252	159	261	199	255	239	298		
40	219	80	214	120	247	160	287	200	213	240	245		

1.4.6 The following data are counts of trypanosomes in the tail blood of rats, successive numbers being counts in different cells of a haemocytometer. Experiments 1 and 2 were done with blood from two different rats on different occasions.

Form the frequency distribution of the number of trypanosomes per cell for each experiment and present these in a form which allows comparison of the two distributions. What do the results suggest about the variability of the method on the two occasions? Illustrate the results by histograms.

Expt. 1															
2	3	2	4	1	2	2	1	1	1	0	2	1	3	2	5
1	4	1	6	0	3	3	3	3	2	2	2	5	0	7	4
3	3	4	5	1	3	5	4	1	6	1	3	1	13	6	3
9	2	8	3	5	5	3	17	9	3	5	7	5	2	0	4
4	4	4	4	1	0	4	1	5	11	4	5	8	3	1	8
6	8	6	2	9	2	13	4	4	5	6	3	2	2	6	6
2	6	4	5	2	6	8	4	9	5	5	3	6	5	2	4
2	2	10	3	7	5	11	6	3	1	2	6	6	3	3	4
4	3	4	5	1	3	5	2	10	5	2	4	1	1	7	1
3	2	3	2	0	1	4	7	1	1	4	0	5	1	2	2
3	2	0	1	5	4	2	11	20	0	6	6	4	3	1	5
9	1	2	2	3	2	3	4	4	3	5	0	7	5	5	2

Expt. 2															
4	6	2	2	2	1	3	5	1	2	2	3	2	4	1	1
5	3	2	6	4	3	3	1	2	6	7	3	5	5	2	2
5	5	6	2	5	1	3	1	9	1	1	2	2	4	1	1
4	4	4	6	1	2	2	1	2	1	0	3	3	4	3	1
4	2	6	2	3	3	7	4	2	6	1	5	2	2	1	9
3	4	4	1	4	6	4	2	5	4	5	4	5	5	6	2
3	1	0	1	5	5	2	2	6	1	3	1	1	1	5	3
1	0	1	5	3	3	6	8	2	0	1	3	6	2	3	5

1.4.7 In a survey of viral hepatitis in an urban population, cases were reported by hospitals, general practitioners and local health authorities. The following table shows the numbers of patients not in hospital and in hospital, subdivided by sex, age and hepatitis B antigen (HBsAG) status.

Obtain summary tables to show how the proportion of patients who are in hospital varies with age, sex and HBsAG status. Comment on the differences revealed.

	HBsAG Positive				HBsAG Negative			
	Not in hospital		In hospital		Not in hospital		In hospital	
Age (yr)	Male	Female	Male	Female	Male	Female	Male	Female
0–14	43	42	25	9	0	0	0	0
15–29	41	39	39	20	18	10	16	7
≥30	48	25	21	10	17	3	18	4

Source: M.Sc. Social Medicine, L.S.H.T.M., 1976.

1.5 MEANS AND OTHER MEASURES OF LOCATION

1.5.1 The data in the table show the distribution of stay in hospital of children under 15 with hypertrophy of tonsils and adenoids with mention of operation, in 4 selected hospital groups, 1960.

Calculate the mean, median and mode duration of stay in each hospital group. Comment on the differences between these three measures and on the differences between the hospital groups.

Hospital group	Duration of stay (days)											Total
	0	1	2	3	4	5	6	7	8	9	10	
A	–	–	16	113	36	5	4	2	1	–	1	178
B	–	1	1	2	2	–	27	–	–	–	–	33
C	–	–	12	33	20	28	35	7	1	4	6	146
D	–	97	6	2	6	28	11	27	2	1	4	184

Source: Heasman M.A. (1964) *Lancet*, **2**, 539.

1.5.2 The table below gives some of the results of a study of the size of reactions to the Mitsuda test (Lepromin) in three groups of children. The children in the first group had been vaccinated at birth with B.C.G. via the oral route and in the second group via the intradermal route whilst the children in the third group had not been vaccinated with B.C.G.

For each group of children calculate the mean, median and mode of the diameters of the reactions. Does the approximate relationship

$$\text{Mode} - \text{Median} = 2 (\text{Median} - \text{Mean})$$

hold for these data?

Diameter of reaction (mm)	Number of children		
	B.C.G. oral	B.C.G. intradermal	No B.C.G. vaccination
1	–	2	7
2	–	3	2
3	36	55	39
4	22	22	–
5	29	42	9
6	18	15	2
7	10	4	–
8	8	4	2
9	3	–	–
10	3	2	–
11	–	–	–
12	3	–	–
13	–	–	–
14	2	1	–
15	1	–	–
16	1	–	–
Total no. children	136	150	61

Source: Azulay R.D. *et al.* (1971) *Internat. J. Leprosy*, **39**, 508.

1.5.3 Mites fed on rats (cotton rat: *Sigmodon hispidus*) infected with the filarial worm *Litomosoides carinii* were later dissected and the number of microfilaria in each mite was counted. The results from dissections of 50 mites are presented in the table below.

Find the mean, median and mode of these counts and comment on the differences between these measures of position.

What are the advantages and disadvantages of the mean, median and mode for describing distributions?

Number of microfilaria per mite									
3	3	1	8	0	7	2	0	10	15
3	19	1	2	42	3	4	7	0	9
0	18	4	6	6	10	1	1	9	14
5	7	5	14	20	6	1	2	14	3
3	5	1	4	3	7	15	7	2	3

1.5.4 The data in the table below show the cumulative percentage distributions of age at marriage (last birthday) for a sample of women in the municipality of San Antonio Illotenango, Guatemala, by birth cohort.

Draw graphs of the four cumulative distributions and estimate the median age at marriage for the four cohorts of women.

Age at marriage	pre–1925 N = 61	1925–34 N = 83	1935–44 N = 90	1945–54 N = 106
	%	%	%	%
9–10	3·4	6·0	5·6	9·6
11–12	6·9	13·3	18·0	21·1
13–14	39·7	27·7	38·2	39·4
15–16	58·6	56·6	68·5	73·1
17–18	63·8	74·7	77·5	90·3
19–20	74·1	80·7	85·4	98·8
21–22	79·3	86·7	89·9	99·0
23–24	82·8	88·0	95·5	100
25–26	87·9	90·4	97·7	
27–28	89·7	92·8	97·7	
29–30	93·1	96·4	98·8	
>30	100	100	100	

Source: Scholl T.O., Odell M.E. & Johnston F.E. (1976) *Ann. Hum. Biol.* **3**, 1, 23.

1.6 MEASURES OF VARIATION

1.6.1 Calculate the mean and standard deviation of the skinfold thicknesses, x, given in exercise 1.4.4 and verify that approximately 95% of the observations are included in the interval mean $\pm$ 2 standard deviations. [$\Sigma x = 1,705 \cdot 5$, $\Sigma x^2 = 27,073 \cdot 47$]

1.6.2 For each group of children calculate the variance and standard deviation of the diameters of reaction to the Mitsuda test from the frequency distributions given in exercise 1.5.2.

1.6.3.   In a trial to assess the value of antitoxin in the treatment of tetanus, a treated group (antitoxin) is compared with a control group (no antitoxin). The allocation of patients to these groups was random and the ages last birthday of the patients are given below. Draw curves of the cumulative relative frequency distributions of age in the two groups separately. Use your curves to estimate the median age and the inter-quartile range for each group.

Antitoxin (A)		No Antitoxin (N)	
41	16	18	33
28	28	24	20
35	27	19	39
40	20	12	36
30	17	29	30
27	12	14	60
50	12	18	17
30	16	18	27
9	20	50	33
40	10	16	14
30	11	14	10
18	20	52	60
31	50	16	12
14	29	40	24
25	24	30	12
27	14	40	10
16	17	40	60
36	25	27	27
25	10	20	8
40	24		
	22		

1.6.4 The data in the table relate to the district of Kigezi, Uganda for the two years 1959–1960.

Calculate for each series the range, mean and standard deviation. Which series shows relatively the largest variation and which the least?

Month	Rainfall (inches)	Mean temperature (°F)	Mean relative humidity at 9 a.m. (%)
January	1·45	72·1	78
February	1·44	72·5	78
March	2·69	72·1	78
April	5·15	72·6	77
May	7·46	73·3	79
June	0·73	73·2	85
July	0·51	72·8	72
August	5·17	71·9	78
September	4·20	71·4	78
October	4·08	71·7	78
November	6·68	71·6	78
December	2·77	71·6	79

CHAPTER 2

PROBABILITY

2.2 PROBABILITY CALCULATIONS

2.2.1 A survey of a Costa Rican community for internal parasites involved a faecal examination of a large sample of the people. Part of the data are summarized in the table below.

If a person were selected at random from this community, what is the probability that he or she is:
(a) Between 15 and 19 years of age?
(b) Less than 15 years of age?
(c) Between 15 and 29 years of age?
(d) Between 15 and 19 years of age, and infected with hookworm?
(e) Between 15 and 29 years of age, and infected with hookworm?
(f) Between 15 and 29 years of age, but not infected with hookworm?
(g) Infected with hookworm?
(h) What is the probability that a person aged between 15 and 29 years is infected with hookworm?

Age group (years)	Proportion of population in age group	Proportion of sample infected with hookworm
0–4	0·20	0·09
5–9	0·18	0·25
10–14	0·14	0·31
15–19	0·09	0·62
20–29	0·13	0·49
30–39	0·10	0·41
40–49	0·07	0·41
50–59	0·04	0·40
60 +	0·05	0·28

Source: Hunter G.W. *et al.* (1965) *Rev. Biol. Trop.* **13,** 123.

2.2.2 For many purposes a baby is said to be premature if its birth weight is $5\frac{1}{2}$ lb or less. Using the data in exercise 1.4.1 calculate (a) the probability that a baby born in South-West England in 1965, is recorded as premature. (b) The recorded birth weight which is exceeded with probability 0·025. (c) The recorded birth weight which is exceeded with probability 0·975.

2.2.3 In a wild population of some *Anopheles* species, 20% of the female mosquitoes are infected with *Plasmodium* spp. Random samples are taken from the population, dissected and examined for Plasmodia. Assume that only female mosquitoes are included in the sample:

(a) In a random sample of 1, what is the probability that the mosquito is infected?
(b) In a random sample of 2, what is the probability that *both* are infected?
(c) In a random sample of 5, what is the probability that 4 or 5 are infected?
(d) In a random sample of 10, what is the probability that at least one will be infected?

2.3 PROBABILITY DISTRIBUTIONS

2.3.1 There are details of the sequence of the sexes of 7,745 families of 4 children recorded in the archives of the Genealogical Society of the Church of Jesus Christ of Latter Day Saints at Salt Lake City, Utah, which are shown below. (*M* indicates a male child and *F* a female child.)

(a) Estimate the probability distribution of these sex sequences in this population.
(b) Estimate the probability distribution of the number of male children, *x*, in these families of four children.
(c) Estimate the probability, π, of a male child in this population and hence, on the assumption that *x* is a binomial variable, calculate the corresponding binomial probability distribution.

Sequence	Frequency	Sequence	Frequency
MMMM	537	MFFM	526
MMMF	549	FMFM	498
MMFM	514	FFMM	490
MFMM	523	MFFF	429
FMMM	467	FMFF	451
MMFF	497	FFMF	456
MFMF	486	FFFM	441
FMMF	473	FFFF	408

Source: Greenberg R.A. & White C. *Proceedings of the 5th International Biometric Conference*, Cambridge. September 10–14, 1963.

2.4 EXPECTATION

2.4.1 Refer to exercise **2.3.1**.

(a) Estimate the expected value of *x*, the number of male children in these families of four children.
(b) Estimate $E(x-\mu)^2$.
(c) Estimate the variance of *x* on the assumption that *x* is distributed binomially.

2.4.2 Random sampling numbers are a sequence of digits between zero and nine, such that the ten digits have an equal and independent probability of occurring at any position in the sequence. (See, for example, Table A6 in Statistical Methods in Medical Research.) What is the mean and variance of random sampling numbers?

2.5 THE BINOMIAL DISTRIBUTION

2.5.1 A suspension of *Leishmania* organisms is prepared and it is found that when a certain quantity is inoculated into mice, 25% of the mice become infected. If three mice are inoculated independently, what are the probabilities that:
   (a) no mice;
   (b) one mouse;
   (c) two mice;
   (d) all three mice become infected?

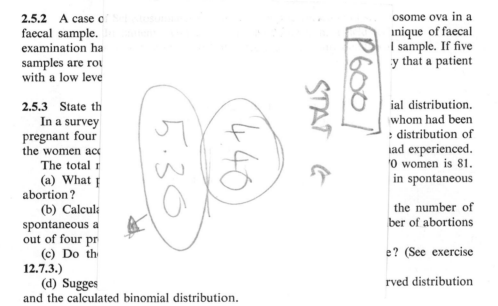

2.5.2 A case o ... osome ova in a faecal sample. ... inique of faecal examination ha ... l sample. If five samples are rou ... y that a patient with a low leve ...

2.5.3 State th ... ial distribution.
   In a survey ... whom had been pregnant four ... e distribution of the women acc ... ad experienced.
   The total r ... 0 women is 81.
   (a) What p ... in spontaneous abortion?
   (b) Calcula ... the number of spontaneous a ... ber of abortions out of four pr ...
   (c) Do th ... e? (See exercise **12.7.3.**)
   (d) Sugges ... rved distribution and the calculated binomial distribution.

	Number of spontaneous abortions				
	0	1	2	3	4
Number of women	24	28	7	5	6

Source: Doyle P. (1974) M.Sc. dissertation, L.S.H.T.M.

2.5.4 Each of 50 chickens was inoculated with exactly 6 ova of *Heterakis gallinarum*. One month later the chickens were killed and 90 adult worms were recovered from the 300 ova. The distribution of the number of recovered worms per chicken is shown below. If the probability of survival from ova to adult worm were equal for all ova and the same in each chicken, the number of surviving worms per host should follow a binomial distribution with $n = 6$ and estimated probability of survival $90/300 = 0.30$. Calculate the frequency distribution expected assuming the binomial model.

Number of worms per chicken	Observed number of chickens
0	9
1	12
2	14
3	11
4	3
5	1
6	0
Total	50

2.6 THE POISSON DISTRIBUTION

2.6.1 The data below (frequency distributions of the observed numbers of anencephalics (stillbirths and infant deaths) in each month compared with expected numbers based on the Poisson distribution, 1956–66), are some of the results of a study of secular and seasonal variations in the incidence of anencephalus in Belfast and four Scottish cities 1956–1966. Verify the expected distribution of cases per month assuming a Poisson distribution with the given means. Do the observed and expected distributions appear to agree well? What does this imply about the seasonal variation in the incidence of anencephalus?

No. of cases per month	Belfast		Glasgow		Edinburgh		Dundee		Aberdeen	
	Obs.	Exp.	Obs.	Exp.	Obs.	Exp.	Obs.	Exp.	Obs.	Exp.
0	7	6·84	1	0·29	18	18·41	48	47·60	82	80·06
1	18	20·25	1	1·75	42	36·26	48	48·68	38	40·03
2	33	29·97	8	5·37	34	35·72	24	24·89	9	10·01
3	32	29·57	15	10·98	18	23·46	10	8·49	2 } 1·91	
4	20	21·88	16	16·84	11	11·55	1 } 2·34		1 }	
5	11	12·95	12	20·67	6	4·55	1 }			
6	3	6·39	25	21·14	0 } 2·05					
7	6	2·70	14	18·53	2 }					
8	2	1·45	15	14·22	1 }					
9			11	9·69						
10			7	5·95						
11			3 } 6·56							
12			2 }							
13			– }							
14			– }							
15			2 }							
Mean	2·96		6·14		1·97		1·02		0·50	
Variance	3·07		7·51		2·39		1·04		0·57	

Source: Elwood J.H. & MacKenzie G. (1971) *Brit. J. prev. soc. Med.* **25**, 17.

2.6.2 A large volume of a suspension of virulent organisms is diluted to a mean concentration of one organism per 0·1 ml. Assuming the organisms are randomly distributed in the suspension and that any one organism will cause an infection in a recipient laboratory animal, what proportion of animals will become infected if 0·1 ml is inoculated into a large number of laboratory animals?

2.6.3 The distribution of *Trypanosoma musculi* in a thin blood film is shown below.
If the trypanosomes were randomly distributed over the oil-immersion fields the distribution of trypanosomes per field should be Poisson. Calculate the frequency distribution of trypanosomes per field assuming they follow a Poisson distribution. Do the observed and theoretical frequency distributions appear to agree well?

Number of trypanosomes per oil-immersion field	Observed number of oil-immersion fields
0	16
1	38
2	30
3	10
4	4
5	1
6	1
7	0

2.6.4 A maternity hospital in London has, on average, 7,200 deliveries per year of which 1·5% are stillborn. What (approximately) is the mean and standard deviation of the number of stillbirths occurring in the hospital per month?

2.6.5 A large survey of over 100,000 births in South Wales during the period 1956–1962 gave an incidence rate for spina bifida of 4·12 per 1,000 births. What is the probability of observing in a random sample of 50 births:
(a) No cases.
(b) One case.
(c) Two cases.
(d) More than two cases.

2.7   THE NORMAL (OR GAUSSIAN) DISTRIBUTION

2.7.1   The iodine content of a tin of salt is stated to be between 433 μg and 753 μg. Assuming that the iodine content is a normally distributed random variable and that it lies between the given limits with probability 0·94 and below the lower limit with probability 0·01, find the probability that the iodine content exceeds:

(a) 500 μg.
(b) 700 μg.
(B.Sc. in Pure Science, University of Durham, July, 1962.)

2.7.2   The data below show the frequency distribution of the 18,645 live birth weights recorded by Pethybridge *et al.* (see exercise **1.4.1**). Draw a cumulative relative frequency curve for the data and estimate the proportion of live birth weights under 5 lb 8 oz. The mean and standard deviation of the birth weights are 118·0 and 19·8 oz respectively. Draw a normal cumulative relative frequency curve with the same mean and standard deviation. What proportion of birth weights would be less than 5 lb 8 oz if the birth weights were normally distributed?

Distribution of live birth weights

Weight, lb	Frequency	Weight, lb	Frequency
0–	3	8–	4305
1–	40	9–	1365
2–	82	10–	240
3–	126	11–	39
4–	364	12–	2
5–	1182	13–	0
6–	4173	14–	1
7–	6723	15–	0
		Total	18,645

Adapted from Pethybridge R.J., Ashford J.R. & Fryer J.G. (1974) *Brit. J. prev. soc. Med.* **28**, 10.

2.7.3 When red blood cells from a patient with *Plasmodium vivax* malaria are examined with a microscope it is found that the mean and standard deviation of the maximum diameter of uninfected red blood cells are 7·6 and 0·9 microns respectively, while for infected cells the mean and standard deviation of the maximum diameter are 9·6 and 1·0 microns respectively. Assuming that the maximum diameters of uninfected and infected cells are normally distributed about their respective means:

    (a) What proportions of uninfected cells would have maximum diameters:
        (i) Greater than 9·4 microns?
        (ii) Greater than 9·6 microns?
    (b) What proportions of infected cells would have maximum diameters:
        (i) Less than 9·4 microns?
        (ii) Less than 7·6 microns?
    (c) Suppose 20% of the cells are infected, i.e. a 20% parasitaemia in this patient. What percentage of all cells will have maximum diameters in excess of 9·0 microns?

2.7.4 The following distribution of haemoglobin levels was obtained from a sample of 711 boys. The mean and standard deviation were estimated to be 95·1 and 9·2 respectively.

Draw a histogram of the relative frequency distribution and plot the cumulative relative frequency curve. Use your curve to find the haemoglobin value, below which
    (a) 5%;
    (b) 30%;
    (c) 70%;
    (d) 95%;
of the sample lie. Compare these with the corresponding values for a normal distribution with the same mean and standard deviation.

Haemoglobin %	Frequency	Relative frequency
60–	1	0·14
65–	1	0·14
70–	4	0·56
75–	21	2·95
80–	58	8·16
85–	114	16·03
90–	171	24·05
95–	159	22·36
100–	94	13·22
105–	47	6·61
110–	15	2·11
115–	21	2·95
120–	4	0·56
125–130	1	0·14
	711	99·98

CHAPTER 3

SAMPLING

3.2 THE SAMPLING ERROR OF A MEAN

3.2.1 The mean and standard deviation of the maximum diameters of uninfected erythrocytes is $\mu = 7\cdot6$ microns and $\sigma = 0\cdot9$ microns. (See exercise **2.7.3**.)

(a) Assuming these maximum diameters are approximately normally distributed, sketch the frequency curve of the maximum diameters of these erythrocytes.

(b) Suppose the maximum diameters of a sample of 30 of these erythrocytes is to be measured. What is the expected value of the mean of these 30 measurements?

(c) What is the standard error of the mean maximum diameter in repeated samples of 30 erythrocites?

(d) Sketch the frequency curve of such repeated sample means.

3.2.2 The following observations of systolic blood pressure in mm were obtained from a random sample of men from a population.

>98, 160, 136, 128, 130, 114, 123, 134, 128, 107.
>123, 125, 129, 132, 154, 115, 126, 132, 136, 130.

The standard deviation of these observations is 13·91 mm.

Estimate the standard error of the mean on the 3 different assumptions that these observations were a simple random sample from:

(a) a finite population of 100 men;

(b) a finite population of 1,000 men;

(c) a finite population of 1,000,000 men.

3.2.3 A dental epidemiologist wishes to estimate the mean weekly consumption of sweets among children of a given age in his area. After devising a scheme which enables him to determine the sweet consumption of a child during a week, he does a pilot survey and finds that the standard deviation of the weekly sweet consumption is about 3 ounces. He considers taking a random sample of either 25 children, or 100 children, or 625 children for the main survey. Estimate the standard error of the sample mean for each of these three sample sizes. How do these standard errors explain why large samples are more reliable than small samples?

3.2.4 The data of exercise **1.4.5** are the sprayable surface areas of 250 houses in an African village. The mean and standard deviation of the sprayable surface areas are 251·75 and 36·76 square feet respectively.

(a) Between what limits of sprayable surface area would you expect 95% of the houses?

(b) What percentage of the 250 houses actually have sprayable surface areas outside these limits?

3.3   THE SAMPLING ERROR OF A PROPORTION

3.3.1   Resistance to dieldrin (0·4%, one hour exposure) in *Anopheles farauti* is deter-mined by a single dominant gene. Thus 25% of the progeny of a parental population of *Anopheles farauti* all of which are heterozygous at this locus should be susceptible to dieldrin. The progeny are tested for dieldrin resistance in lots of 50 mosquitoes.

(a) Express, in terms of the standard error, the variation in the percentage of sus-ceptibles which would be expected in repeated lots of 50 mosquitoes.

(b) What is the standard error of the percentage of resistant progeny in samples of 50 mosquitoes?

(c) Find a level which the percentage of resistant mosquitoes would exceed in only 5% of such lots.

3.3.2   The following observations of diastolic blood pressure were obtained from a sample of men.

Estimate:

(a) The proportion of men in the population with a diastolic blood pressure greater than 95 mm.

(b) The standard error of this proportion on the 2 different assumptions that these observations were a simple random sample from:

(i) A finite population of 1,000 men.

(ii) A finite population of 1,000,000 men.

94	94	82	100	112	110	84	78	92	112
94	92	86	84	90	72	88	92	88	84
98	98	84	90	90	70	80	90	80	106
74	95	100	94	84	70	102	92	84	80
84	86	98	82	80	88	80	84	100	86

3.3.3   In a population of children of school entering age, a proportion, 0·2, possess the sickle cell trait.

(a) What is the standard error of the percentage of sicklers in repeated samples of 200 children from this population?

(b) Find a level which this percentage would exceed in only 5% of repeated samples of this size.

CHAPTER 4

STATISTICAL INFERENCE

4.2 and 4.3 SIGNIFICANCE TESTS ON A SAMPLE MEAN AND INTERVAL ESTIMATION OF A MEAN

4.2.1 The mean level of prothrombin in the normal population is known to be 20·0 mg/100 ml of plasma and the standard deviation is 4 mg/100 ml. A sample of 40 patients showing vitamin K deficiency has a mean prothrombin level of 18·50 mg/100 ml.

(a) How reasonable is it to conclude that the true mean for patients with vitamin K deficiency is the same as that for the normal population?

(b) Within what limits would the mean prothrombin level be expected to lie for all patients with vitamin K deficiency? (i.e. give 95% confidence limits).

4.2.2 In an investigation of the relationship between general health and oral pathology, the mean DMFS score (a count of Decayed, Missing and Filled tooth Surfaces in an individual's mouth) of all Naval Aviation Cadets was found to be 27·2 with standard deviation 15·5. In 121 cadets who made 5 or more dispensary visits, the mean DMFS score was 31·1. If it is assumed that these 121 subjects represented the cadets in poorest general health, is there any evidence that poor general health is associated with an increased DMFS score?
Source: Manhold J.H. & Izard C.E. (1954) *Science*, **120**, 892.

4.2.3 Armitage, P. (Statistical Methods in Medical Research, section 3.2) describes an experiment in which a computer took 2,000 samples of 5 random digits. The mean value of the 2,000 sample means was 4·5391. The sampling distribution of repeated sample means of 5 random digits is shown theoretically to have a mean of 4·5 and standard error 1·28. Is there any strong evidence to suggest that random digits generated by the computer do not have a mean of 4·5?

4.2.4 Two nematode species, *G. primum* and *G. secundum*, are described as having ova which are morphologically very similar but with different size distributions. Ova of species *Primum* are said to have an average length of more than 50 microns while ova of species *Secundum* have an average length of less than 50 microns.

Twelve ova of this morphological type are found in the faeces of a patient. The lengths of the ova are in microns:

37·2	38·6	41·2	42·4	44·8	46·3
48·1	49·4	49·7	50·4	51·6	52.7

Do these data provide evidence as to which of the two species is affecting the patient?

4.4 INFERENCES FROM PROPORTIONS

4.4.1 Dr J. Bryan (personal communication) recently examined the theory that resistance to dieldrin (0·4%, one hour exposure) is due to a single dominant gene in *Anopheles farauti*. Homozygous resistants (RR) were crossed with homozygous susceptibles (rr), to give a heterozygous F1 population. The F1 mosquitoes were then back-crossed to the homozygous susceptible strain. According to the theory of single gene determination, the percentage of the progeny of this back-cross which should be susceptible to dieldrin is 50%. Of 465 back-cross progeny exposed to the dieldrin dose, 264 or 56·77% died. Is this percentage significantly different to the percentage predicted by the genetic model?

4.4.2 In an investigation into the teratogenic properties of a drug a control group (i.e. not receiving the drug) of 85 pregnant rats was observed. Of the 85 litters produced, 12 contained at least one malformed offspring. Find 95% confidence limits for the true proportion of such litters in the population of rats from which the 85 are assumed to have been sampled.

4.4.3 A large number of mites are placed on a cotton rat with microfilarial infection. After a certain time 50 mites are dissected and 10 found to be infected. Assuming that the dissected mites were effectively a random sample of the whole population, give 95% confidence limits for the percentage of mites infected in the whole population.

4.4.4 In a report of adult dental health in England and Wales, of a sample of 262 women aged 25–34, 7·6% were edentulous, whereas in the U.S.A., 6·1% of women of this age were edentulous. Calculate a 95% confidence interval for the proportion of women aged 25–34 who were edentulous in England and Wales at that time. Deduce from the confidence interval whether the difference between the sample proportion, 7·6% and the value 6·1% is significant at the 5% level.
Source: Gray P.G. *et al.* (1970) Adult Dental Health in England and Wales in 1968, London H.M.S.O.

4.4.5 The 'spleen rate' in a population is of great interest to malaria epidemiologists. MacDonald (*The Epidemiology and control of malaria, 1957*) defines this as: 'The percentage of children aged from 2 to 10 inclusive, in whom the spleen is palpable when in the standing position.'
    Suppose you palpate the abdomen of 85 randomly selected children, aged 2–10, in a malarious area. In 12 of the children the spleen is palpable.
    Calculate 95% and 99% confidence intervals for the true 'spleen rate' in the population from which these children were drawn.

4.4.6 You examine 500 erythrocytes in a thin film from a sick water buffalo, and note that 84 contain *Babesia* sp. parasites. Calculate 90% and 95% confidence intervals for the parasitaemia level in this animal, assuming that the blood examined can be considered a random sample of the animal's total blood.

4.4.7 A standard dose of the parasite *Schistosoma mansoni* was transmitted to 20 rats. After a period of 4 weeks the rats were killed and the number of adult parasites was counted. The total number of parasites found in the 20 rats was 36 of which 27 were males.

(a) What is the estimated proportion of male parasites in a large population of rats of the same strain?

(b) What can be said about the limits within which the population proportion would be likely to lie?

4.6 COMPARISON OF TWO MEANS

4.6.1 A certain drug is to be tested for its effect on blood pressure. Twelve male patients have their diastolic blood pressure measured before and after receiving the drug with the results shown below (in mmHg).

(a) Do these results indicate that the drug may have an effect on diastolic blood pressure?

(b) Calculate a 95% confidence interval for the average effect in patients of this type.

Patient	BP before	BP after	Patient	BP before	BP after
1	120	125	7	140	146
2	124	126	8	135	133
3	130	138	9	126	127
4	118	117	10	130	135
5	140	143	11	126	126
6	128	128	12	127	131

Source: (B.Sc. in Pure Science, University of Durham, 1960).

4.6.2 The following data represent the additional hours of sleep in ten patients due to the use of drug A rather than drug B.

(a) Investigate whether the soporific effects of the two drugs are likely to be equal on the average.

(b) Calculate a 95% confidence interval for the true mean increase in sleep due to the use of drug A rather than drug B.

+1·2	+2·4	+1·3	0·0	+1·0	+1·8	+0·8	-4·6	+1·4	+1·3

Source: 'Student' (1908) *Biometrika*, **VI**, 1–25.

4.6.3 Of interest is the effect of a certain treatment on the body temperature of guinea pigs. The rectal temperatures of ten guinea pigs was measured at noon on the day before they were treated, and again at noon, on the day following the treatment. The primary data are given below:

Animal number	Temperature on day before treatment	Temperature on day after treatment
1	38·1	38·9
2	38·4	38·6
3	38·3	38·2
4	38·2	38·2
5	38·2	39·4
6	37·9	38·5
7	38·7	38·3
8	38·6	38·4
9	38·0	38·8
10	38·2	38·7

(a) Is there evidence that the treatment has any effect on the body temperature of guinea pigs?

(b) Calculate a 95% confidence interval for the true average change in temperature.

4.6.4 The following are the results of a biometric study of weights of kidneys in a series of autopsies of males in a pathology department of a hospital in Africa.

(a) Estimate the average difference in weight between the left and right kidneys in the hospital population from which this sample was taken and its standard error.

(b) Can the sample mean difference be reasonably explained in terms of sampling error?

Kidney weights (grammes)	
170	150
155	145
140	105
115	100
235	222
125	115
130	120
145	105
105	125
145	135
155	150
110	125
140	150
145	140
120	90
130	120
105	100
95	100
100	90
125	125

Source: Diploma in Tropical Public Health, 1973, University of London.

4.6.5 A study of blood alcohol levels (mg/100 ml) at post mortem examination from traffic accident victims involved taking one blood sample from the leg, A, and another from the heart, B. The results were:

Case	A	B	Case	A	B
1	44	44	11	265	277
2	265	269	12	27	39
3	250	256	13	68	84
4	153	154	14	230	228
5	88	83	15	180	187
6	180	185	16	149	155
7	35	36	17	286	290
8	494	502	18	72	80
9	249	249	19	39	50
10	204	208	20	272	290

Do these results indicate that in general blood alcohol levels may differ between samples taken from the leg and the heart?

4.6.6 The following results were obtained in a study of the changes in creatine phosphate during the chromatolysis of Nissl bodies in the anterior horns of the spinal cord following section of the sciatic nerve. The left sciatic nerve of 10 monkeys was sectioned. The phosphocreatine content of the anterior horns of the cervical cord was determined for both the regenerating left side and the normal right side for each animal.

Test the significance of the mean difference in phosphocreatine content between the regenerating and normal cells.

	Phosphocreatine in the anterior horn of monkey spinal cord (mg P per 100 g tissue)	
Animal	Regenerating left	Normal right
1	5·6	7·4
2	4·3	8·0
3	12·5	10·9
4	8·9	20·6
5	4·6	16·8
6	6·1	31·8
7	5·0	15·9
8	18·0	22·6
9	9·8	17·6
10	10·6	15·2

4.6.7 The following data show the distribution of live birth weights recorded at Macha Mission Hospital in Zambia for the years 1965 and 1975. Has there been a significant change in mean birth weight at the hospital during this 10–year period?

Birth weight (Kilos)	Number of babies 1965	1975	Birth weight (Kilos)	Number of babies 1965	1975
1·6–	1	0	2·9–	35	31
1·7–	0	0	3·0–	28	39
1·8–	2	4	3·1–	28	26
1·9–	2	1	3·2–	35	22
2·0–	8	1	3·3–	15	21
2·1–	2	2	3·4–	24	17
2·2–	8	2	3·5–	5	21
2·3–	9	7	3·6–	14	13
2·4–	14	9	3·7–	6	8
2·5–	5	14	3·8–	7	9
2·6–	22	14	3·9–	1	10
2·7–	39	23	4·0–4·1	1	2
2·8–	20	30			
			Total	331	326

Source: Byer D.E. Unpublished data.

4.6.8 In a study of the age of menarche in women in the U.S.A., the following distributions were observed for samples of women aged 21–30 and 31–40 years. The ages at menarche quoted are to the nearest whole number of years. Test the hypothesis that there is no difference in the average age of menarche between the two groups of women. Calculate a 95% confidence interval for the true difference.

Age at menarche	Women aged 31–40 yrs	Women aged 21–30 yrs
10	0	3
11	2	11
12	8	28
13	14	23
14	27	12
15	5	1
16	8	0
17	1	0
18	1	0
Total	66	78

Source: adapted from Damon A. et al. (1969) Hum. Biol. 41, 161.

4.6.9 The following data show the abrasiveness of two brush-on denture cleaners, A and B, measured by weight loss in grammes.

A:	0·0102	0·0110	0·0096	0·0098	0·0099
	0·0105	0·0112	0·0095	0·0101	0·0118
B:	0·0096	0·0085	0·0090	0·0098	
	0·0107	0·0090	0·0095	0·0099	

Do these data provide evidence that one of these denture cleaners is more abrasive than the other? If so, calculate a 95% confidence interval for the true average difference.

4.6.10 The following are some of the results of a study of the size of reactions to the Mitsuda test (lepromin). One group of children, O, had been vaccinated with B.C.G. at birth with an oral vaccine, the other group, I, being vaccinated intra-dermally. Do these results present evidence that the reactions to the Mitsuda test are greater (as measured by the diameter of infiltration) on the average in one group rather than the other?

Diameter of infiltration (mm)	Group O frequency	Group I frequency
1	0	2
2	0	3
3	36	55
4	22	22
5	29	42
6	18	15
7	10	4
8	8	4
9	3	0
10	3	2
11	0	0
12	3	0
13	0	0
14	2	1
15	1	0
16	1	0
Total No. children	136	150

Source: Azulay R.D. *et al.* (1971) *Internat. J. Leprosy*, **39**, 2, 508–521.

4.6.11 Of interest is the effect of a low dose of cambendazole on *Trichinella spiralis* infections in mice. Sixteen mice were infected with equal numbers of *Trichinella* larvae and then randomly allocated to two groups. The first group of 8 mice received cambendazole (10 mg/kg) sixty hours after infection. The other 8 mice received no treatment. After one week all the mice were killed and the following numbers of adult worms recovered from their intestines:

Untreated mice:	51	55	62	63	68	71	75	79
Treated mice:	44	47	49	53	57	60	62	67

What can be concluded about the effectiveness of cambendazole (10 mg/kg) for treating *Trichinella spiralis* infections in mice?

4.6.12 In a trial to compare a stannous fluoride dentifrice A, with a commercially available fluoride free dentrifice D, 260 children received A and 289 received D for a 3-year period. The mean DMFS increments (the number of new *D*ecayed *M*issing and *F*illed tooth *S*urfaces) were 9·78 with standard deviation 7·51 for A and 12·83 with standard deviation 8·31 for D. Is this good evidence that, in general, one of these dentrifices is better than the other at reducing tooth decay? If so, within what limits would the average annual difference in DMFS increment be expected to be?

Source: Slack G.L. *et al.* (1971) *Br. dent. J.* **130**, 154.

4.6.13 The following data show the mean number of decayed missing and filled teeth (DMF score) in two samples of 3 to 4-year-old children according to their average weekly sweet consumption.

	No. children	Mean DMF	Standard deviation
Sweet consumption < 8 oz	34	2·32	0·98
Sweet consumption ≥ 8 oz	19	3·63	1·10

Is here strong evidence to indicate that, in general, there is an association between DMF score and sweet consumption? Calculate a 95% confidence interval for the difference in DMF score between the two groups of children.

Source: Mansbridge J.N. Proceedings of the Conference on Dental Epidemiology, London Hospital Medical College, 16–18 November, 1966.

4.6.14 In a randomized trial, 111 pregnant women had elective induction of labour between 39 and 40 weeks and 117 controls were managed expectantly until 41 weeks. The blood loss after delivery was measured for all the women with the following results:

	Induction group	Control group
Number of patients	111	117
Blood loss after vaginal delivery (ml) mean	185	233
Standard deviation	139	150

Obtain a pooled estimate of the variance and investigate whether the mean blood loss differs significantly between the two groups.

4.6.15 In the assay of digitalis, a tincture of digitalis is infused intravenously at a slow constant rate into the heart of an anaesthetized cat until the cat dies. The experiment is stopped and the total dose injected (the 'just fatal' dose) is read. The data following are log doses ($+0.5$) for a standard tincture (tested on 10 cats) and an unknown (tested on 8 cats). Test whether the mean fatal log dose is different for the two tinctures, and give 95% confidence limits for the difference between the mean logs.

Standard	Unknown
0·077	0·186
0·156	0·316
0·163	0·344
0·194	0·348
0·221	0·350
0·251	0·389
0·256	0·423
0·260	0·476
0·289	
0·359	

4.6.16   A study of immunoglobulin levels in mycetoma patients in the Sudan involved 22 patients to be compared with 22 normal individuals. The levels of IgG recorded for the 22 mycetoma patients are shown below. The mean level for the normal individuals was calculated to be 1,477 mg/100 ml before the data for this group was lost overboard from a punt on the River Nile. Use the data below to estimate the within group variance and hence perform a 't' test to investigate the significance of the difference between the mean levels of IgG in mycetoma patients and normals.

IgG levels (mg/100 ml) in 22 mycetoma patients				
1,047	1,135	1,350	1,122	1,345
1,377	1,375	804	1,062	1,204
1,210	1,067	1,032	1,002	1,053
1,103	907	960	960	936
1,270	1,230			

4.7   COMPARISON OF TWO PROPORTIONS

4.7.1   A new schizonticidal drug is tested against chloroquine sulphate in equivalent doses, with particular reference to its speed of action. The criterion of success for the purposes of the trial is complete clearance of all asexual parasites from the blood within 36 hours, as judged by a 10-minute thick film examination. The results of the trial are as follows:

Drug	Total number of cases	Number of cases with 36-hour clearance
Chloroquine sulphate	184	129
New drug	103	80

(a) Calculate the proportion of cases with 36-hour clearance for each of the two drugs.

(b) What is the difference between the two proportions and its standard error?

(c) Within what limits do you expect the true difference to lie?

(d) Do these limits enable you to draw any conclusion as to whether one of these drugs is better than the other?

4.7.2 Eighty cockroaches are divided into eight groups of ten roaches apiece, and exposed to DDT. Three groups (30 roaches in all) are subjected to a dose of 11 μg/g; and five groups (50 roaches) are subjected to 20 μg/g. The numbers of roaches surviving in each of the groups are as follows:

Dose (μg/g)	Survivors (out of 10)				
11	10	8	9		
20	6	6	7	7	7

(a) Assuming that the results at a given dose level are sufficiently similar to be pooled, would you say that there is a difference in the true survival rates at the two doses?

(b) Within what limits would it be fairly safe to estimate the true difference in survival rates? (i.e. calculate a 95% confidence interval for the true difference).

4.7.3 An experiment was designed to investigate whether the smoke of cigarette papers is a carcinogenic agent of lung tumours. In this experiment 74 mice were used, of which 38 served as experimental and 36 as control animals. The experimental mice were placed in the experimental cage and the controls in the control cage of the smoking machine. The machine was set to smoke 108 cigarette papers per day, six days per week for one year.

At the end of the experiment the animals were sacrificed. There were 13 tumours in the experimental and 11 in the control mice.

The author states: 'There is a very slight preponderance of tumours in the experimental over the control mice which is not significant by statistical analysis. . . . The results of this experiment indicate that cigarette paper has little or no effect on the generation of lung tumours in albino mice.'

(a) Perform an appropriate statistical analysis to check the first of these conclusions. What is your conclusion from the analysis?

(b) Do you agree with the second statement in the author's conclusion?

4.7.4 In a study of the response to typed and mimeographed letters in a survey using postal questionnaires the following results were obtained:

Response rate for typed and mimeographed first letters

Type of letter	No. sent	Useful replies	% useful replies
Mimeographed	189	108	57·1
Typed	192	110	57·3
Total	381	218	57·2

Response rate for first letters personally signed and first letters signed on a stencil

Type of signature	No. sent	Useful replies	% Useful replies
Stencil	50	30	60·0
Personal	51	25	49·0
Total	101	55	54·5

The author's comment:

(a) . . . mimeographed covering letters are just as likely to elicit useful replies as individually typed letters.

(b). . . a personally signed letter was no more likely to elicit a useful response than one with a mimeographed signature the response rates being 49% and 60% respectively. Letters were sent to relatively small numbers of surgeons, so that the difference in rates may be attributed to chance.

To what extent do you agree with these comments?

Source: Kelsey J.L. & Acheson R.M. (1971) *Brit. J. prev. soc. Med.* **25,** 177.

4.7.5 In a study of the cariostatic properties of dentrifices 423 children were issued with dentrifice A and 408 were issued with dentifrice D. After 3 years, 163 of the children on A and 119 of the children on D had withdrawn from the trial. The authors suggest that the main reason for withdrawal from the trial was because the children disliked the taste of the dentrifices. Do these data indicate that one of the dentrifices is disliked more than the other?

Source: Slack G.L. *et al.* (1971) *Brit. dent. J.* **130,** 154.

4.7.6 In a case-control study, 317 patients suffering from endometrial carcinoma were individually matched with 317 other cancer patients in a hospital and the use of oestrogen in the six months prior to diagnosis was determined. The results were:

		Controls	
		Oestrogen used	Oestrogen not used
Cases	Oestrogen used	39	113
	Oestrogen not used	15	150

Use McNemar's test to investigate the significance of the association between oestrogen use and endometrial carcinoma.

4.8 FOURFOLD TABLES AND χ^2 TESTS

4.8.1 From each of 509 vaginal swabs taken at a London veneral disease clinic, isolation of *Candida albicans* and culture of *Trichomonas vaginalis* were attempted.

There were 347 swabs negative for both *Candida* and *Trichomonas*. Candida was isolated from 7 of the 44 swabs positive for *Trichomonas*.

Construct a 2 × 2 table and investigate the evidence of an association between Candidiasis and Trichomoniasis.

4.8.2 It is suggested that eating piping hot food, served at say 150°F and a moment later taking a cold drink or vice versa, exposes the teeth to thermal shock. One effect of thermal shock on vitreous materials is to induce small cracks which accelerate mechanical breakdown. In the case of teeth, such small cracks could lead to dental decay. In an experiment, 50 extracted healthy teeth, free from fillings were given thermal shocks by repeatedly immersing them in boiling water and ice water. Fifty similar control teeth were gently boiled avoiding thermal shock. The teeth were then subjected to a crushing test. Of the 50 teeth which had been given the thermal shocks, 21 broke. Of the 50 control teeth 11 broke. Do these results indicate an association between thermal shock and the mechanical strength of teeth?
Source: Pohl D.G. & Pohl H.A. (1954) *Science*, **120**, 807–808.

4.8.3 In an investigation into the relationship between the incidence of colds at different periods of time a random sample of 100 persons was selected from a certain population. During two different periods of time,

    42 were attacked in both periods,
    11 were attacked in the first period, but not in the second period,
    19 were not attacked in either period.

Construct a 2 × 2 table and investigate whether those attacked in the first period are more or less likely to be attacked in the second period than those who were not attacked in the first.

Do this using both the test for independence in a contingency table and the test for the difference between two proportions.

4.8.4 In a randomized trial 111 pregnant women had elective induction of labour between 39 and 40 weeks and 117 controls were managed expectantly until 41 weeks. The patients with elective induction were stated to have had significantly less meconium staining in labour than the control patients. The results were:

	Induction group	Control group
Number of patients	111	117
Meconium staining	1	13

Use Fisher's exact test to verify the author's conclusion.

Source: Adapted from M.Sc. Social Medicine, September 1975.

4.8.5 A report states: 'Comparison of the 90 normotensive patients with the 10 patients with hypotension shows that only 3·3% of the former group died as against 30% of the latter'. Construct a 2 × 2 contingency table and test the significance of blood pressure as a prognostic sign.
(a) Using χ^2 without continuity correction
(b) Using χ^2 with continuity correction
(c) Using Fisher's exact test

4.8.6 In a trial of diabetic therapy, patients were either treated with Phenformin or a placebo. The numbers of patients and deaths from cardiovascular causes were as follows.

	Treatment group		
	Phenformin	Placebo	Total
Cardiovascular deaths	26	2	28
Not cardiovascular deaths	178	62	240
Total	204	64	268

Use Fisher's exact test to investigate the difference in cardiovascular mortality between the Phenformin and Placebo treatment groups.

Source: Gray R.H. (1973) *Med. J. Aust.* **1**, 594–596.

4.9 COMPARISON OF TWO COUNTS

4.9.1 An airline recorded 48 'near-misses' on its flights in 1974 but 62 in 1975. Did the number of 'near-misses' increase significantly between these two years? Estimate a 95% confidence interval for the percentage increase in near misses between 1974 and 1975.

D

4.9.2   The data below show the numbers of sand-flies (*Lutzomyia disponeta*) caught in light traps set three feet and thirty-five feet above ground at a site in Eastern Panama. At each height, do the counts of male and female flies differ significantly?

	Height above ground	
	3 ft	35 ft
No. males caught	173	125
No. females caught	150	73

Source: Christensen H.A. *et al.* (1972) *Ann. trop. Med. Parasit.* **66**, 1, 55–66.

4.9.3   The number of isolations of *Salmonella boydii* in 216 Indian children suffering with diarrhoea and 138 non-diarrhoeal children are shown below:

	Diarrhoeal children	Non-diarrhoeal children
S. boydii isolated	6	3
S. boydii not isolated	210	135

Use the Poisson approximation to investigate whether there is a significant difference between the two proportions of children from whom this organism was isolated.

Source: Sanyal S.C. *et al.* (1977) *J. trop. Med. Hyg.* **80**, 1, 2–8.

4.10   COMPARISON OF TWO VARIANCES

4.10.1   Repeated analyses of a certain brand of food have established that its mean nitrogen content is 1·81 g% with standard deviation 0·025 g%. Two new laboratory workers A and B obtain the following results in 10 repeated analyses of the same food.

Worker A	Worker B
1·73	1·85
1·75	1·86
1·80	1·80
1·83	1·83
1·79	1·87
1·88	1·85
1·85	1·90
1·79	1·84
1·78	1·84
1·80	1·86

For each worker, is there evidence that:
(a) his experimental technique is not up to the general laboratory standard?
(b) his results are biased?

4.10.2   The diagnosis of *Schistosoma haematobium* infections is usually based on finding the characteristic ova in the urine of the patient. Counts of the number of ova per urine sample give an indication of the number of worms present and hence the severity of the infection. It is thought that the sensitivity of this test varies with the time of collection of the urine sample.

The following data show the number of ova (in thousands) passed in the urine at different times of the day by the same patient.

a.m.	p.m.
6·9	23·3
2·7	10·8
6·2	16·9
2·6	20·0
2·2	18·2
1·3	20·5
5·5	11·8
2·2	6·8
1·2	13·2

Such variation in egg output makes the estimation of the numbers of worms rather difficult. Do these data present evidence that the variance of the egg output is less at one time rather than the other?

4.10.3   The weight gains of uninfected rats are to be compared with the weight gains of rats infected with a coccidian parasite. Six week weight gains (in grammes) for the rats are shown below:

Uninfected:	136	146	104	119	124	161	107
	83	113	129	97	123		
Infected:	70	118	101	85	107	132	94

It is proposed to make the comparison using the two sample 't' test. Do these data indicate that the assumption of equality of variance is likely to be invalid?

CHAPTER 5

REGRESSION AND CORRELATION

5.2 LINEAR REGRESSION

5.2.1 The following data show the percentage of young children caries free before and after fluoridation of the water supply in some North American cities.

% caries free			
Before F. (x)	After F. (y)	Before F. (x)	After F. (y)
18·2	49·2	25·0	23·0
21·9	30·0	13·0	17·0
5·2	16·0	76·0	79·0
20·4	47·8	59·0	66·0
2·8	3·4	25·6	46·8
21·0	16·8	50·4	84·9
11·3	10·7	41·2	65·2
6·1	5·7	21·0	52·0

$\Sigma x = 418 \cdot 1$, $\Sigma x^2 = 17{,}252 \cdot 75$, $\Sigma y = 613 \cdot 5$, $\Sigma y^2 = 34{,}070 \cdot 55$
$\Sigma xy = 23{,}078 \cdot 04$, $n = 16$.

(a) Draw a scatter diagram to show the association, if any, between x and y.

(b) Calculate the equation of the regression line of y on x and draw the line on your scatter diagram.

5.2.2 Fifteen chickens were fed embryonated ova of the nematode *Heterakis galli-narum*. Fifty days later, total daily egg output counts were made on 24 hour faeces collections from each of the birds. The chickens were then killed, and the number of female worms in their intestinal tracts (caeca) counted. The actual data are summarized below:

Chicken number	x Number of female *Heterakis*	y Estimated number of *Heterakis* ova passed in faeces over 24 hours
1	2	1,343
2	3	3,067
3	10	15,752
4	24	15,821
5	9	8,762
6	23	19,985
7	12	7,851
8	14	11,704
9	12	13,989
10	1	661
11	4	4,794
12	2	476
13	12	7,067
14	1	346
15	10	8,278

$$n = 15 \qquad \Sigma x^2 = 2,049$$
$$\Sigma x = 139 \qquad \Sigma y^2 = 1,522,359,912$$
$$\Sigma y = 119,896 \qquad \Sigma xy = 1,702,279$$

(a) Draw a scatter diagram to show the association, if any, between the number of female worms present and the total daily egg output.

(b) Calculate the equation of the regression line of y on x and draw the line on your diagram.

(c) Interpret the regression coefficient (slope) of the line in terms of the daily egg production per female *Heterakis*.

(d) Should the line go through the origin (the point $x = 0$, $y = 0$)? Does it?

(e) Comment on the assumptions underlying this method of calculating the daily egg output of a nematode.

5.2.3 The relationship between malaria parasitaemia and pyrexia was investigated by measuring parasitaemia levels and body temperatures in patients infected with Plasmodium species.

Parasitaemia levels are measured by the estimated number of parasites per mm^3 of blood. Body temperature was measured on a haemotothermic scale in which the $10°$ between $95°F$ and $105°F$ are divided into 100 equal units.

Parasitaemia level, x	Body temperature, y
1,500	84
1,400	101
580	97
440	102
430	76
260	76
256	54
232	46
150	44
133	34
100	34
83	20

(a) Plot the data on a scatter diagram.

(b) Does the relationship between parasitaemia and body temperature appear linear?

(c) Calculate the equation of the regression line of body temperature on parasitaemia level for that part of the scatter diagram for which the relationship appears linear.

5.3 CORRELATION

5.3.1 The following data give the pre-war averages of the net food supply, x and the infant mortality rates, y for certain selected countries:

Country	No. calories per person per day x	Infant mortality rate per 1,000 y	Country	No. calories per person per day x	Infant mortality rate per 1,000 y
Argentina	2,730	98·8	Iceland	3,160	42·4
Australia	3,300	39·1	India	1,970	161·6
Austria	2,990	87·4	Ireland	3,390	69·6
Belgium	3,000	83·1	Italy	2,510	102·7
Burma	2,080	202·1	Japan	2,180	60·6
Canada	3,070	67·4	New Zealand	3,260	32·2
Ceylon	1,920	182·8	Norway	3,160	40·5
Chile	2,240	240·8	Netherlands	3,010	37·4
Columbia	1,860	155·6	Poland	2,710	139·4
Cuba	2,610	116·8	Sweden	3,210	43·3
Denmark	3,420	64·2	Switzerland	3,110	45·3
Egypt	2,450	162·9	U.K.	3,100	55·3
France	2,880	66·1	U.S.A.	3,150	53·2
Germany	2,960	63·3	Uruguay	2,380	94·1
Greece	2,600	113·4			

Draw a scatter diagram to show the association, if any, between the average daily number of calories per person and the infant mortality rate. Calculate the correlation coefficient. Does a plentiful food supply reduce infant mortality? (See also exercise **9.1.1.**)

Source: United Nations (1954) *Population Studies*, Number **13**, New York.

5.3.2 The following data taken from the U.K. Annual Abstract of Statistics 1970 show the number of post-graduate awards in medical sciences, x, and the death rate per million from tuberculosis, y, for the years 1959–1969.

Year	Number of awards, x	Tuberculosis D.R./10^6, y	Year	Number of awards, x	Tuberculosis D.R./10^6, y
1959	277	83	1965	750	47
1960	318	74	1966	738	48
1961	382	71	1967	849	42
1962	441	65	1968	932	43
1963	486	62	1969	976	38
1964	597	52			

$n = 11$, $\Sigma x = 6{,}746$, $\Sigma x^2 = 4{,}760{,}008$, $\Sigma y = 625$, $\Sigma xy = 346{,}982$, $\Sigma y^2 = 37{,}749$ $(\Sigma x)^2/n = 4{,}137{,}137\cdot81$, $(\Sigma y)^2/n = 35{,}511\cdot36$, $(\Sigma x)(\Sigma y)/n = 383{,}295\cdot45$

Draw a scatter diagram to show the association between x and y. Calculate the (product-moment) correlation coefficient of x and y. How many post-graduate awards in medical sciences would be needed in order to reduce the tuberculosis death rate to zero? Explain the reasons for your answer.

5.3.3 The data below show the consumption of alcohol in litres per year, per person aged more than 14 years and the death rate per 100,000 population from cirrhosis and alcoholism in selected countries. Draw a scatter diagram to show the association, if any, between these variables and calculate the correlation coefficient. (See also exercises **9.1.2.** and **13.4.2.**)

Country	Consumption of alcohol (litres per person per year)	Death rate per 100,000 from cirrhosis and alcoholism
France	24·7	46·1
Italy	15·2	23·6
West Germany	12·3	23·7
Australia	10·9	7·0
Belgium	10·8	12·3
U.S.A.	9·9	14·2
Canada	8·3	7·4
England and Wales	7·2	3·0
Sweden	6·6	7·2
Japan	5·8	10·6
Netherlands	5·7	3·7
Ireland	5·6	3·4
Norway	4·2	4·3
Finland	3·9	3·6
Israel	3·1	5·4

5.3.4 In a study of the relationship between length, and egg production, of female *Enterobius vermicularis* (human 'threadworm', or 'piuworm') the data, based on 14 worms, and the published diagram, are shown below:

Worm number	Length in mm (x)	Number of ova contained in worm (y)
1	6·7	4,672
2	7·0	7,698
3	7·5	4,902
4	8·1	12,782
5	8·8	8,790
6	8·8	8,706
7	9·0	10,507
8	9·0	8,506
9	9·0	11,810
10	9·2	14,703
11	9·3	14,816
12	9·4	6,345
13	9·4	11,024
14	9·7	14,451

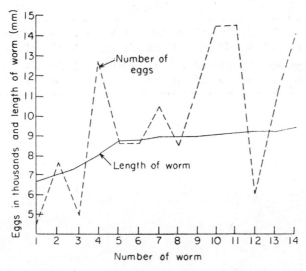

Suggest a better way of presenting this data, and investigate the correlation between the two variables concerned.

5.3.5 The following are the heights (measured to the nearest 2 cm) and weights (measured to the nearest kg) of 80 male and 34 female second-year undergraduate medical students.

(a) Draw scatter diagrams to show the association between heights and weights separately for males and females but on the same diagram.

(b) Calculate the correlation coefficient of height and weight for the males and females separately. Retain the values of Σx, Σx^2, Σy, Σy^2 and Σxy.

(c) Calculate the correlation coefficient of height and weight for males and females together.

(d) Comment on the possible effects on the correlation coefficient of combining two or more groups of data.

MALES

Height	162	168	170	170	170	170	170	170	172	174	174	174	174	174	174	174
Weight	65	65	58	59	67	68	74	81	66	61	64	65	67	68	70	71
Height	174	176	176	176	176	176	178	178	178	178	178	178	178	178	180	180
Weight	84	63	64	65	74	81	66	69	71	71	72	73	75	77	70	72
Height	180	180	180	180	180	180	182	182	182	182	182	182	182	182	182	182
Weight	75	76	77	78	80	82	63	66	72	72	72	73	73	75	79	79
Height	182	182	184	184	184	184	184	184	184	184	186	186	186	186	186	186
Weight	82	83	65	68	75	76	78	78	81	85	66	68	68	69	76	77
Height	186	186	188	188	188	188	188	190	190	190	190	192	192	194	194	198
Weight	80	81	59	64	70	80	85	70	71	72	72	75	79	73	82	76

FEMALES

Height	152	154	156	156	158	158	160	160	162	162	162	164	164	164	164	164	166
Weight	52	48	50	56	47	53	48	59	52	55	55	48	55	55	56	60	56
Height	166	166	168	168	168	168	168	168	170	170	172	172	174	174	178	178	180
Weight	65	66	55	60	61	62	64	66	53	61	60	68	57	71	67	70	65

5.3.6 The data below show the mean annual mortality for males aged 45–64 during 1958-1964 and the calcium ion concentration in drinking water for 61 large towns of England and Wales.

(a) Draw a scatter diagram to show the association between these two variables.

(b) Calculate the correlation coefficient.

(c) Calculate the linear regression of mortality on calcium content.

Towns	Mortality per 100,000 (y)	Calcium ppm (x)	Towns	Mortality per 100,000 (y)	Calcium ppm (x)
Bath	1,247	105	Newcastle	1,702	44
Birkenhead	1,668	17	Northampton	1,309	59
Birmingham	1,466	5	Norwich	1,259	133
Blackburn	1,800	14	Nottingham	1,427	27
Blackpool	1,609	18	Oldham	1,724	6
Bolton	1,558	10	Oxford	1,175	107
Bootle	1,807	15	Plymouth	1,486	5
Bournemouth	1,299	78	Portsmouth	1,456	90
Bradford	1,637	10	Preston	1,696	6
Brighton	1,359	84	Reading	1,236	101
Bristol	1,392	73	Rochdale	1,711	13
Burnley	1,755	12	Rotherham	1,444	14
Coventry	1,307	78	St Helens	1,591	49
Croydon	1,254	96	Salford	1,987	8
Darlington	1,491	20	Sheffield	1,495	14
Derby	1,555	39	Southampton	1,369	68
Doncaster	1,428	39	Southend	1,257	50
East Ham	1,318	122	Southport	1,587	75
Exeter	1,260	21	Southshields	1,713	71
Gateshead	1,723	44	Stockport	1,557	13
Grimsby	1,379	94	Stoke	1,640	57
Halifax	1,742	8	Sunderland	1,709	71
Huddersfield	1,574	9	Wallasey	1,625	20
Ipswich	1,096	138	Walsall	1,527	60
Hull	1,569	91	West Bromwich	1,627	53
Leeds	1,591	16	West Ham	1,486	122
Leicester	1,402	37	Wolverhampton	1,485	81
Liverpool	1,772	15	York	1,378	71
Manchester	1,828	8	Cardiff	1,519	21
Middlesborough	1,704	26	Newport	1,581	14
			Swansea	1,625	13

5.4 SAMPLING ERRORS IN REGRESSION AND CORRELATION

5.4.1 Refer to exercise **5.2.1**.

(a) Predict the percentage of young children who would be caries free in a particular town where before fluoridation 60% were caries free. What is the standard error of this predicted value?

(b) What is the standard error of the estimated regression coefficient b?

(c) Test the hypothesis that the true regression coefficient, β, is unity. What would this imply about the percentage of young children caries free before and after fluoridation?

5.4.2 Refer to exercise **5.3.1**. Test the hypothesis that there is no linear association between the net food supply and the infant mortality rate.

5.4.3 Refer to exercise **5.3.3**. Test the hypothesis that there is no linear association between consumption of alcohol and mortality from cirrhosis and alcoholism.

5.4.4 Refer to exercise **5.3.6**.

(a) Test the hypothesis that there is no linear association between male mortality at ages 45–64 and calcium content of drinking water.

(b) For a town with 100 ppm calcium ion predict the male mortality at ages 45–64.

(c) Calculate a 95% confidence interval for the predicted value.

(d) Calculate a confidence belt to include 95% of towns and draw it on the scatter diagram. What percentage of towns are actually included within the confidence belt?

5.4.5 The data show the malaria epidemic index (x) and the November spleen rate (y) for the years 1914–1943 in the Punjab, India. The malaria epidemic index is calculated by dividing the average monthly fever mortality from October to December by the corresponding average of the previous April to July of each year. The November spleen rate is the proportion of subjects sampled from the population in November with palpable spleens.

Year	Malaria epidemic index (x)	November spleen rate (y)
1914	1·32	16·5
1915	1·10	11·1
1916	1·76	12·4
1917	2·46	16·2
1918	0·47	12·3
1919	1·51	12·1
1920	0·83	8·7
1921	1·28	11·1
1922	1·38	9·8
1923	1·93	15·7
1924	1·49	15·1
1925	1·40	15·5
1926	1·83	17·3
1927	1·00	15·8
1928	0·99	11·4
1929	1·79	16·2
1930	1·23	15·6
1931	1·33	13·0
1932	1·16	11·1
1933	2·11	18·5
1934	1·17	12·8
1935	1·07	10·8
1936	1·01	9·2
1937	0·97	6·7
1938	0·79	5·3
1939	0·98	6·0
1940	1·25	8·5
1941	1·28	9·5
1942	2·54	16·2
1943	1·48	13·6

(a) Test the hypothesis that the slope of the regression line of y on x is zero.

(b) Test the hypothesis that the correlation between the malaria index and the November spleen rate is zero. How does this compare with the result of your test in part (a)?

(c) Find the 95% confidence interval for the predicted *mean* spleen rate when the malaria index is 1·0, 1·5 and 2·0.

(d) Plot a scatter diagram, draw the estimated regression line and, using your results from (c), sketch out the 95% confidence belt for the true regression line.

(e) A particular year has a malaria index of 1·5. Find the 95% confidence interval for predicting its spleen rate.

(f) The table below shows the difference between the observed spleen rate and that calculated from the regression equation for each year. These differences are called the 'residuals'. What is their correlation with x and standard deviation? (No computation required.)

(g) Examine the residuals by year. Do they show any pattern? What does this suggest?

(h) A physician estimates that the November spleen rate is now 4·0. Derive a regression estimate of the expected malaria index and give 95% confidence limits for the value the index might have taken this year.

(i) From your plot of the data, question (g) above, and generally say why you would view the results of question (h) with caution.

Year	x	y	Predicted spleen rate Y	Residual $y-Y$
1914	1·32	16·5	12·3	4·2
1915	1·10	11·1	11·2	−0·1
1916	1·76	12·4	14·4	−2·0
1917	2·46	16·2	17·9	−1·7
1918	0·47	12·3	8·1	4·2
1919	1·51	12·1	13·2	−1·1
1920	0·83	8·7	9·8	−1·1
1921	1·28	11·1	12·1	−1·0
1922	1·38	9·8	12·6	−2·8
1923	1·93	15·7	15·3	0·4
1924	1·49	15·1	13·1	2·0
1925	1·40	15·5	12·7	2·8
1926	1·83	17·3	14·8	2·5
1927	1·00	15·8	10·7	5·1
1928	0·99	11·4	10·6	0·8
1929	1·79	16·3	14·6	1·7
1930	1·23	15·6	11·8	3·8
1931	1·33	13·0	12·3	0·7
1932	1·16	11·1	11·5	−0·4
1933	2·11	18·5	16·1	2·4
1934	1·17	12·8	11·5	1·3
1935	1·07	10·8	11·0	−0·2
1936	1·01	9·2	10·7	−1·5
1937	0·97	6·7	10·5	−3·8
1938	0·79	5·3	9·7	−4·4

1939	0·98	6·0	10·6	−4·6
1940	1·25	8·5	11·9	−3·4
1941	1·28	9·5	12·1	−2·6
1942	2·54	18·2	18·3	−2·1
1943	1·48	13·6	13·0	0·6

CHAPTER 6

THE PLANNING OF STATISTICAL

INVESTIGATIONS

6.2 THE PLANNING OF SURVEYS: ESTIMATION OF POPULATION PARAMETERS

6.2.1 A stratified sample of general hospitals (stratified by size) with a variable sampling fraction is drawn in each of three regions. The table shows, for each hospital in the sample, the number of patients discharged (including deaths) in a given week with a diagnosis of cancer of the lip.

Size group (beds)	1–50	51–200	201–500	501–
Sampling fraction	1/20	1/10	1/5	1/3
No. of hospitals in sample	10	16	11	7
Region I	1, 0, 2	3, 4, 2, 1	6, 1, 0	12, 5, 8
Region II	0, 0, 1	0, 5, 0, 3, 2	4, 0	6
Region III	0, 0, 0, 0	4, 0, 0, 0, 0, 3, 1	2, 1, 0, 7, 5, 4	10, 8, 4

(a) Estimate the total number of patients discharged in the week with a diagnosis of cancer of the lip, and the proportion of hospitals discharging at least one patient with this diagnosis.

(b) What are the estimated standard errors of these quantities?

6.2.2 The table below gives information on absences from work because of accidents during a year in a factory. Calculate the standard errors of the estimates of the total days lost when,

(a) a simple random sample of 200 persons is taken from the whole population;
(b) a stratified random sample of 100 men and 100 women is taken;
(c) the total sample of 200 is optimally allocated to the two strata.

	Men	Women	Total
Number of persons	500	450	950
Mean days lost from accidents	8	2	5·16
Estimated variance of days lost	67	5	42

6.2.3 A school dental officer wishes to estimate the total number of primary school children in his district who require dental treatment by conducting a sample survey. From his training in dental public health he knows that the proportion, p, of children requiring treatment increases with age roughly as follows:

Age (years):	4–5	6–7	8–9	10–11
p	0·05	0·07	0·15	0·20

He believes there are roughly equal numbers of children in each age group. How should he allocate his total sample to the age groups in order to minimize the standard error of the estimated total number of children requiring treatment?

6.5   THE SIZE OF A STATISTICAL INVESTIGATION

6.5.1 Expiratory flow rate, EFR, measured in litres per minute is often used as a measure of respiratory function. As a result of extensive experience with a variety of subjects it is known that the standard deviation, σ, of repeated EFR readings on the same subject is about 8 litres/min irrespective of the particular subject used.

N patients are to be used to determine the effect of a bronchodilator, A, on the EFR. The EFR is to be measured twice on each patient, once after treatment with an inert substance and once after A has been given. The order of the two tests is to be randomized.

(a) How large must N be for a mean difference of 5 litres/min to be significant at the 5% level?

(b) If you wanted to be sure that a *true* mean difference of 5 litres/min would not be missed in 97·5% of trials, would you increase the size of N? If so, what should N be?

6.5.2 In a housing survey a random sample of dwellings is to be taken from each of two regions, A and B, and the mean number of rooms per dwelling is to be measured in each sample. A pilot sample of dwellings is taken from each region and from these samples the standard deviation of the number of rooms per dwelling, within regions, is estimated as 1·5.

(a) In the main survey the sample size in each region is to be n dwellings. How large should n be to make it possible to estimate the difference between A and B in the mean number of rooms per dwelling to within $\pm 0\cdot 1$? (This can be interpreted as meaning that the 95% confidence interval for the difference has width 0·2.)

(b) Suppose that we want to be particularly careful not to miss a difference of 0·2 rooms per dwelling, if such a difference exists. (We can interpret this as meaning that we want a probability of 0·95 of getting a difference significant at the 5% level.) How large should n be for this purpose?

E

6.5.3 A survey of 1,000 schoolchildren aged 7–8 years in a rural tropical district estimated the prevalence of malaria as 20%. A new irrigation scheme is to be introduced to facilitate the growing of cotton and it is considered desirable to monitor malaria prevalence annually to assess the effect of the new scheme. What should be the size of the sample of schoolchildren at the end of the first year to give a 95% chance of observing a true change of (a) 10%, (b) 5% in the prevalence rate, significantly at the 1% level?

What conclusion can you draw from your answer to (b)?

CHAPTER 7

COMPARISON OF SEVERAL GROUPS

7.1 ONE-WAY ANALYSIS OF VARIANCE

7.1.1 The table shows the number of days to death of 31 mice inoculated with three strains of typhoid organism.

(a) Carry out an analysis of variance to test whether the differences between the three means are significant.

(b) Calculate the standard error of each mean using the within-group mean square. What can be said about the ordering of the three groups in terms of time to death?

(c) Do you think the use of the pooled within-group mean square in the calculation of standard errors is justifiable here? If not, what other procedure would you suggest?

| | Strain | |
9D	11C	DSC1
2	8	8
4	7	6
6	5	12
5	8	6
2	4	8
4	7	7
4	6	10
3	10	5
5	9	7
5		11
		9
		3

7.1.2 The cariostatic effects of four dentifrices A, B, C and D were compared by randomly allocating children to dentifrice groups and following them up for a period of 3 years. For each child the response variable, x, was the 3 year DMFS increment, that is, a count of new *D*ecayed *M*issing or *F*illed tooth *S*urfaces. Dentifrices A and C contained stannous fluoride, B contained sodium fluoride while D was fluoride free. The results were:

	\multicolumn{5}{c}{Dentifrice}
	A	B	C	D	Total
No. children	260	279	282	289	1,110
$\bar{x}$	9·78	11·62	10·56	12·83	11·24
Σx	2,543	3,242	2,978	3,708	12,471
Σx^2	39,476	52,690	50,066	67,460	209,692

(a) Construct an analysis of variance table and test for differences between the mean increments.

(b) Use the 'within' mean square to estimate the standard errors of the four group means.

(c) Is the difference between the mean increments of the two stannous fluoride dentifrices A and C significant? If not, combine the two groups and calculate the pooled mean and its standard error.

(d) Do the results provide strong evidence to suggest that the stannous fluoride dentifrices A + C have a different cariostatic effect to the sodium fluoride dentifrice B?

(e) Does the sodium fluoride dentifrice B have a significantly different cariostatic effect to the fluoride free dentifrice D?

(f) Summarize these results.

Source: Slack G.L., Bulman J.S. & Osborn J.F. (1971) *Brit. Dent. J.* **130,** 154–158.

7.1.3 Four groups of mice were given different numbers of daily injections of oestrone and for each mouse was measured the increase in mm of the inter-pubic gap 24 hours after a single injection of relaxin. The results are given below:

Group	\multicolumn{6}{c}{Data}
1	0·15	0·50	0·40	0·40	0·30	
2	1·90	2·30	1·35	1·50	1·40	1·20
3	2·00	2·20	1·20	1·40	2·20	0·50
4	1·50	2·50	2·50	1·50		

Apply a test of significance to examine whether the differing numbers of oestrone injections affect the increase in width, and comment.

7.2 COMPONENTS OF VARIANCE

7.2.1 The following measurements of systolic blood pressure (mmHg) were obtained (a) with a conventional sphygmomanometer and (b) with a new instrument in which the observer presses a button on hearing the appropriate sounds and the reading is subsequently taken from a stationary scale. The same observers were used in both sets of data.

(a) Systolic blood pressure, usual method
Observer

Subject	1	2	3	4	5	Total
1	124	118	120	122	124	608
2	108	104	108	120	108	548
3	130	128	138	116	124	636
4	152	128	132	150	142	704
5	128	124	118	112	142	624
6	126	122	120	120	132	620
7	118	104	118	120	128	588
Total	886	828	854	860	900	4,328

(b) Systolic blood pressure, new method
Observer

Subject	1	2	3	4	5	Total
1	108	116	112	124	114	574
2	96	92	94	104	100	486
3	120	128	130	118	120	616
4	124	128	118	132	132	634
5	110	110	100	98	110	528
6	118	116	110	120	118	582
7	120	102	104	116	120	562
Total	796	792	768	812	814	3,982

The analysis of variance for the two methods yields:

	Sums of squares		Degrees of freedom
	Method (a)	Method (b)	
Between subjects	2,731·89	3,049·37	6
Between observers	454·18	197·03	4
Residual	1,353·82	807·77	24
Total	4,539·89	4,054·17	34

Estimate the components of variance for subjects, observers and residual variation and express these as a percentage of the total variance for each of the two methods.

7.2.2   In a pilot survey of systolic blood pressure in men of a certain age group, a random sample of men was selected from a large population of factory workers and each of these men had his blood pressure recorded on a number of occasions by the same observer. The components of variance were estimated as follows:

$$\text{Between men} \qquad 100\cdot0$$
$$\text{Between occasions} \quad 50\cdot0$$

In the main survey it is intended to take n men and observe each man's blood pressure on r occasions. Calculate the standard error of the estimated mean blood pressure of all men in the population, for the following values of n and r.

	(a)	(b)	(c)
n	100	100	1,000
r	1	10	1

(The sampling fraction can be assumed to be small.)

If 1,000 blood pressure determinations can be made in the survey, is (c) necessarily better than (b)?

7.3 MULTIPLE COMPARISONS

7.3.1   In a study of four antidotes A, B, C and D to three poisons I, II and III, for each antidote-poison combination the mean survival time of four animals is recorded. (See exercise **8.2.1**.) The estimated standard error of any one of the means is $0\cdot0745$ with 36 d.f. For each of the three poisons use the Newman–Keuls procedure to test the significance of the difference between the mean survival times under the four treatments.

Mean survival times

Poison	Treatment			
	A	B	C	D
I	0·4125	0·8800	0·5675	0·6100
II	0·3200	0·8150	0·3750	0·6675
III	0·2100	0·3350	0·2350	0·3250

7.3.2 In a study of the pollution of inland waterways five pike were caught in each of seven localities and the log concentration of copper in the livers of the fish was measured. The results were:

Locality	Log concentration of copper (ppm)				
Windermere	0·187	0·836	0·704	0·938	0·124
Grassmere	0·449	0·769	0·301	0·045	0·846
River Stour	0·628	0·193	0·810	0·000	0·855
Wimbourne St Giles	0·412	0·286	0·497	0·417	0·337
River Avon	0·243	0·258	−0·276	−0·538	0·041
River Leam	0·134	0·281	0·529	0·305	0·459
River Kennett	0·471	0·371	0·297	0·691	0·535

Use the Newman–Keuls method for the multiple comparison of the seven group means. (The within groups variance, $s^2 = 0.0816$.)

7.3.3 It has been suggested that women who excel in track and field sports have more masculine physiques than female non-athletes. In a study, androgyny scores were measured for fifty female athletes and ten non-athlete college students. The androgyny score is defined as ($3 \times$ biacromial breadth–bicristal breadth). The results were:

Athletic category	n	Mean androgyny score
A. Non-athletes	10	79·93
B. Distance runners	10	80·01
C. Sprinters	10	81·98
D. Jumpers and Hurdlers	10	84·95
E. Discus and Javelin	10	86·47
F. Shotputters	10	88·89

The estimated standard error of any group mean is 1·20 with 54 degrees of freedom.

Use the Newman–Keuls method to investigate the significance of differences in the mean androgyny scores of women in the athletic categories.

7.4 COMPARISON OF SEVERAL PROPORTIONS: THE $2 \times k$ CONTINGENCY TABLE

7.4.1 The following data show the results of caries surveys in five towns and also the fluoride content of the drinking water. (See exercise **12.2.2**.)

Area F p.p.m.	Surrey and Essex 0·15	Slough 0·9	Harwich 2·0	Burnham 3·5	West Mersea 5·8	Total
No. children with dental caries	243	83	60	31	39	456
No. children with caries free teeth	16	36	32	31	12	127
No. examined	259	119	92	62	51	583

The data refer to samples of children aged 12–14 only. Do a significance test to determine whether the proportions of children caries free varies from area to area. What does this test reveal about the effect of the fluoride content of the water?

7.4.2 The following results are taken from a randomized trial to compare the effects of an oral hypoglycaemic drug (T), an indistinguishable placebo (P), a standard dose of insulin (IS) and a variable dose of insulin (IV) on patients with adult-onset diabetes, all of whom received additional dietary treatment. The recruitment of patients lasted about 5 years and the follow-up continued for a further 3 years.

Investigate the evidence for a differential rate of mortality in patients receiving these four treatments.

	Treatment			
	P	T	IS	IV
Deaths during follow-up	21	30	20	18
Survivors	179	170	180	182
Total	200	200	200	200

Source: Adapted from M.Sc. Social Medicine, University of London, 1972.

7.4.3 The deaths which occurred during the follow-up described in exercise **7.4.2** were classified as being from cardiovascular causes or other causes as follows:

	Treatment			
Cause of death	P	T	IS	IV
Cardiovascular	10	26	13	12
Other	11	4	7	6
All deaths	21	30	20	18

Do the proportions of deaths from cardiovascular causes differ significantly between the treatment groups?

Source: Adapted from M.Sc. Social Medicine, University of London, 1972.

7.4.4 Pregnancies with retarded intra-uterine growth observed in a clinic were classified as to whether threatened miscarriage occurred and whether the placenta was circumvallate (3 degrees, normal, minor and major) at delivery. (See exercise **12.2.3**.)

	Placenta			
Miscarriage	Normal	Minor	Major	Total
Threatened	10	18	14	42
Not threatened	36	12	8	56
Total	46	30	22	98

Investigate the association between threatened miscarriage and the degree to which the placenta is circumvallate at delivery.

7.5 GENERAL CONTINGENCY TABLES

7.5.1 In a study of the blood groups of blood donors in South-West Scotland, the following distributions were obtained for seven regions. Is there evidence to suggest that the distributions of blood groups differ from region to region?

Blood group	Region				Dee &			
	Eskdale	Annandale	Nithsdale	Urr	Fleet	Cree	Rhinns	Total
A	33	54	98	34	33	38	36	326
B	6	14	35	9	14	9	9	96
O	56	52	115	39	55	79	47	443
AB	5	5	5	8	5	6	7	41
Total	100	125	253	90	107	132	99	906

Source: Mitchell R.J. *et al.* (1976) *Annals of Human Biology*, **3**, 2, 157–171.

7.5.2　In a study of sex maturation in Turkish girls, a sample of 12 to 13-year-old girls were classified by the socio-economic class of their parents and stage of breast development. Stage of breast development was graded from 1 representing elevation of papillae only, a flat chest, to 5 for a mature or near-mature breast.

Number of subjects at various stages of breast development by parental socio-economic class

Socio-economic class of parents	Breast development					Total
	1	2	3	4	5	
1	2	14	28	40	18	102
2	1	21	25	25	9	81
3	1	12	12	12	2	39
4	6	17	34	33	6	96
Total	10	64	99	110	35	318

Notice that the expected frequencies of girls at the first stage of breast development are relatively small.

(a) Use χ^2 to investigate the association between stage of breast development and parental socio-economic class ignoring the problem of the small frequencies.

(b) Combine the first two stages of breast development and recalculate χ^2 to investigate the association.

(c) Are the conclusions reached in (a) and (b) largely similar?

Source: Neyzi O., Alp H. & Orhon A. (1975) *Ann. Hum. Biol.* **2**, 1, 49–59.

7.5.3　During a dental health campaign in Dundee, children were examined without warning and their oral hygiene was graded as: Good, Fair +, Fair −, or Bad. Also the schools they attended were classified by 'social grades' as: Below Average, Average and Above Average. The two-way classification yielded the following results:

Social grade of school	Oral hygiene				Total
	Good	Fair +	Fair −	Bad	
Below average	62	103	57	11	233
Average	50	36	26	7	119
Above average	80	69	18	2	169
Total	192	208	101	20	521

Do these results present evidence of an association between the state of oral hygiene in children and the social grade of the school that they attend?

Source: Finlayson D.A. & Pearson J.C.G. (1967) *Br. Dent. J.* **123**, 535–536.

7.7 COMPARISON OF SEVERAL COUNTS: THE POISSON HETEROGENEITY TEST

7.7.1 In a period of one year, ten workers in a factory doing the same work under the same conditions had the following numbers of accidents:

1	2	2	3	5	6	6	7	8	10

Do these workers show significant differences in accident proneness?

7.7.3 The following are counts of the ova of *Schistosoma mansoni* in equivalent sized portions of a human stool:

369	383	391	473	425	357

Is it likely that the ova are randomly distributed throughout this human stool?

7.7.3 The number of accidents per month in a factory on the day and night shifts during a 10-month period are shown below:

Month	1	2	3	4	5	6	7	8	9	10	Total
Day shift	7	6	8	5	8	8	7	7	7	8	71
Night shift	10	8	7	7	10	8	10	7	8	9	84

Do these data suggest that accidents do not occur randomly on:
  (a) The day shift?
  (b) The night shift?

CHAPTER 8

FURTHER ANALYSIS OF VARIANCE

8.1 TWO-WAY ANALYSIS OF VARIANCE: RANDOMIZED BLOCKS

8.1.1 Refer to exercise **7.2.1**. Verify the given analysis of variance of systolic blood pressures obtained by the two methods.

8.1.2 In a series of assays of pertussis vaccines, three vaccines were tested on each of ten days. The responses given below are estimates of the logarithms of the doses of vaccine (in millions of organisms) required to protect 50% of mice against a subsequent infection with pertussis organisms.

(a) Test whether the differences between days and between vaccines are significant.

(b) The log potency of vaccine A compared with vaccine B is estimated by the difference in the mean responses, $\bar{y}_B - \bar{y}_A$. Calculate 95% confidence limits for the true log potency.

Day	Vaccine A	Vaccine B	C	Total
1	2·64	2·93	2·93	8·50
2	2·00	2·52	2·56	7·08
3	3·04	3·05	3·35	9·44
4	2·07	2·97	2·55	7·59
5	2·54	2·44	2·45	7·43
6	2·76	3·18	3·25	9·19
7	2·03	2·30	2·17	6·50
8	2·20	2·56	2·18	6·94
9	2·38	2·99	2·74	8·11
10	2·42	3·20	3·14	8·76
Total	24·08	28·14	27·32	79·54

$$\Sigma y^2 = 215\cdot4524$$

8.1.3 In a survey of Polish tuberculosis patients a pilot measurement of average weekly dietary energy intake was carried out on 5 patients for one week. The investigators wished to know whether, in the main survey they would get a biased result if they only collected data for weekdays (Monday, Tuesday, Wednesday, Thursday and Friday).

(a) Perform a two-way analysis of variance to investigate whether there are significant differences between patients and between days.

(b) Is there evidence to suggest that the mean dietary energy intake is different on weekdays to that on weekend days?

Patient	Sun.	Mon.	Tues.	Wed.	Thurs.	Fri.	Sat.
			Energy intakes (MJ)				
1	15·2	12·6	10·7	15·5	12·7	9·7	13·8
2	12·5	12·3	12·1	14·0	17·1	9·9	10·2
3	12·8	8·6	13·2	11·4	12·2	7·2	10·9
4	10·1	12·8	13·4	13·5	13·5	11·0	12·8
5	18·0	16·5	18·7	13·5	13·5	12·4	11·9

$$\Sigma y^2 = 5896\cdot82$$

8.2 FACTORIAL DESIGNS

8.2.1 The table below gives the survival times of animals in a 3×4 factorial experiment, the factors being:
(a) three poisons and
(b) four treatments.

Each combination of the two factors is used for four animals, the allocation to animals being completely randomized.

Survival times (unit 10 hr) of animals

Poison	Treatment							
	A		B		C		D	
I	0·31	0·45	0·82	1·10	0·43	0·45	0·45	0·71
	0·46	0·43	0·88	0·72	0·63	0·76	0·66	0·62
II	0·36	0·29	0·92	0·61	0·44	0·35	0·56	1·02
	0·40	0·23	0·49	1·24	0·31	0·40	0·71	0·38
III	0·22	0·21	0·30	0·37	0·23	0·25	0·30	0·36
	0·18	0·23	0·38	0·29	0·24	0·22	0·31	0·33

Without transforming the data (see exercise **11.3.4**) calculate the analysis of variance to test the effects of the two factors and their interaction.

Source: Box G.E.P. & Cox D.R. (1964) *J. R. Statist. Soc. B.* **26**, 211–252.

8.2.2 The data below were part of an investigation into the experimental errors involved in using a photo-electric titration method on an influenza virus preparation. Each of three operators A, B and C performed eight titrations on the same preparation, four titrations in which a single pipette was used for each dilution (single pipette) and four in which a fresh pipette was used for each dilution (multiple pipette).

Operator

A		B		C	
Single pipette	Multiple pipette	Single pipette	Multiple pipette	Single pipette	Multiple pipette
290	282	285	310	269	261
277	255	209	286	331	255
282	233	252	282	266	249
243	251	265	320	289	255

Perform a two-way analysis of variance and test for differences between operators, for differences between methods and the interaction.

8.2.3 The results given below are taken from an assay of vitamin D on rats. There are 4 treatments (2 doses on each of two preparations), and 8 rats from each of 6 litters are allocated randomly to the treatments, so that each treatment is represented twice in each litter. The responses are assessments, by means of the line test on bones, of the antirachitic activity of the vitamin, and are measured on an arbitrary scale from 0 to 12.

Carry out the analysis of variance, with the following sub-division of degrees of freedom.

Litters	5
Treatments	3
⎰ Preparations 1	
⎱ Doses 1	
Prep. × doses 1	
Litters × treatments	15
Residual	24
Total	47

Litter	Standard preparation		Test preparation	
	Low dose	High dose	Low dose	High dose
I	3	4	4	5
	3	7	6	7
II	2	4	4	5
	2	4	5	6
III	2	5	4	5
	3	5	4	5
IV	3	4	4	5
	3	5	5	7
V	3	4	3	6
	3	4	2	5
VI	3	4	3	4
	4	5	6	7

Hint: The residual sum of squares may be calculated conveniently from the difference between replicate readings,

$$\text{i.e.} \quad \frac{(3-3)^2}{2} + \frac{(4-7)^2}{2} + \dots$$

8.3 LATIN SQUARES

8.3.1 The following data are taken from an experiment in which each of four rabbits received four different doses of insulin on four different days. The logarithms of the doses (in units of insulin per kilogram of body weight) were as follows:

$$D_1 \quad 0.32$$
$$D_2 \quad 0.47$$
$$D_3 \quad 0.62$$
$$D_4 \quad 0.77$$

The responses shown in the table are percentage reductions in blood sugar (and were obtained by taking the mean of five readings at successive hourly intervals after injection of insulin).

	Rabbit							
	1		2		3		4	
Day	Dose	B.S.R.	Dose	B.S.R.	Dose	B.S.R.	Dose	B.S.R.
1	D_3	32·7	D_1	11·2	D_2	23·2	D_4	48·1
2	D_2	26·2	D_4	31·8	D_3	28·9	D_1	18·7
3	D_1	−4·0	D_3	14·0	D_4	27·5	D_2	25·6
4	D_4	33·2	D_2	16·5	D_1	21·2	D_3	40·2

(a) Test whether there are significant differences in response due to:
   (i) Differences between rabbits;
   (ii) Different days;
   (iii) Different doses.
(b) Calculate the mean responses at the four doses, and their standard errors.

8.3.2 In an assay of streptomycin, an 18-hour growth of *Staphylococcus aureus* was added in tubes to agar and to this was added the fluid to be assayed. The response was the depth (mm) of the zone of inhibition. However, it was suspected that the time taken to fill the tubes was a source of error. In order to investigate these timing errors, 25 tubes were arranged as a Latin square such that the row numbers show the order in which agar was added to the tubes, while the column numbers are the order in which the fluid was added. There were five concentrations of streptomycin, say A, B, C, D and E. The results were as follows:

		Columns				
		1	2	3	4	5
	1	D 6·7	B 3·7	E 7·6	C 5·5	A 0·8
	2	E 7·9	D 6·8	C 5·3	A 1·3	B 3·3
Rows	3	B 3·7	E 8·2	A 1·0	D 6·6	C 5·1
	4	A 0·8	C 5·2	D 6·7	B 3·7	E 7·6
	5	C 5·3	A 0·8	B 3·6	E 7·5	D 6·6

Do these results imply that errors due to the time to fill the tubes with agar (rows) and fluid (columns) are significant?

Source: Adapted from Mitchison D.A. & Spicer C.C. (1949) *J. gen. Microbiol.* **3**, 2, 184–203.

8.4 OTHER INCOMPLETE DESIGNS

8.4.1 In a balanced incomplete block design comparing seven thermometers, only blocks of three thermometers could be simultaneously maintained at the same temperature. The results given below are expressed in hundredths of a degree above 25°C.

Thermometers	Temperatures							Totals
	1	2	3	4	5	6	7	
A	40	32	81					153
B			108	84	84			276
C	66			54		70		190
D			62			43	21	126
E	34				55		44	133
F		92			109	82		283
G		28		28			27	83
Totals	140	152	251	166	248	195	92	1,244

The sum of the squares of all 21 values in 88,750.

Obtain the sum of squares between thermometers, adjusted for temperatures, and test it for significance.

Source: B.Sc. in Pure Science, University of Newcastle-upon-Tyne (1964).

F

8.5 SPLIT-UNIT DESIGNS

8.5.1 Plasma testosterone concentrations were investigated in pairs of men who were closely matched for age, height, weight, marital status and occupation. One man of each pair was a life-long non-smoker while the other smoked at least 30 cigarettes daily. Two specimens were collected with an interval of 7 days. During this interval none of the men smoked.

Plasma testosterone (ng/ml)

		Specimen 1	Specimen 2
Pair 1	Smoker	5·4	7·2
	Non-smoker	7·9	8·0
Pair 2	Smoker	4·8	5·9
	Non-smoker	7·7	7·5
Pair 3	Smoker	4·3	6·2
	Non-smoker	8·1	8·3
Pair 4	Smoker	6·1	7·2
	Non-smoker	7·4	8·0
Pair 5	Smoker	5·8	7·2
	Non-smoker	6·9	7·0
Pair 6	Smoker	4·5	6·1
	Non-smoker	6·8	6·7

Construct an analysis of variance table for this data showing the sum of squares between men broken into contributions due to between pairs and between smoking groups, and the within men sum of squares broken into contributions due to specimens and the smoking × specimen interaction.

Source: Briggs M.H. (1973) *Med. J. Aust.*, **1**, 616–617.

8.5.2 A study was designed to assess four techniques of measuring blood pressure in infants and children. The four techniques were auscultation (A), Doppler (D), flush (F) and palpatation (P) and observations of systolic blood pressure using these techniques were compared with the intra-arterial measurement which is considered accurate but unsuitable for routine use. The data below show the differences (in mmHg) between the intra-arterial measurement and the measurements made by the four techniques A, D, F and P. Observations were made on 21 children by both a nurse and a doctor.

(a) Perform an analysis of variance splitting the degrees of freedom as follows. (The uncorrected total sum of squares is 91,772.)

Source of variation	df
Subjects	20
Observers	1
Error	20
Techniques	3
T × O interaction	3
Error	120
Total	167

(b) Calculate the mean value of the differences and its standard error for each of the four techniques.

Observer	Nurse					Doctor					Subject total
Technique	A	D	F	P	Total	A	D	F	P	Total	
Subject											
1	−10	−10	−45	−15	−80	−5	0	−45	−25	−75	−155
2	−15	−15	−45	−25	−100	5	5	−25	−10	−25	−125
3	−10	−18	−45	−10	−83	−15	−15	−40	−10	−80	−163
4	−5	−4	−65	−26	−100	−15	−15	−60	−20	−110	−210
5	−10	−15	−40	−20	−85	−10	−4	−40	−30	−84	−169
6	−5	0	−40	−10	−55	−10	−5	−35	−10	−60	−115
7	2	−2	−30	0	−30	0	0	−25	−10	−35	−65
8	0	5	−55	−10	−60	−5	−5	−65	−5	−80	−140
9	7	5	−48	2	−34	5	0	−42	−2	−39	−73
10	−7	3	−42	0	−46	5	5	−35	−5	−30	−76
11	0	8	−30	−5	−27	10	5	−25	0	−10	−37
12	−10	−5	−50	−15	−80	0	−5	−40	−15	−60	−140
13	6	5	−40	−12	−41	−5	−2	−40	−10	−57	−98
14	5	10	−20	−15	−20	0	5	−20	−15	−30	−50
15	0	−5	−32	−5	−42	5	5	−35	−5	−30	−72
16	−5	0	−55	−14	−74	0	0	−40	−10	−50	−124

8.5.2—*contd.*

17	0	−5	−42	−5	−52	−5	−10	−45	−5	−65	−117
18	0	0	−40	−5	−45	−5	−10	−45	−5	−65	−110
19	5	−2	−58	−10	−65	−10	0	−60	−20	−90	−155
20	−2	2	−55	−5	−60	−24	−26	−45	−20	−115	−175
21	−5	−5	−45	−5	−60	−5	0	−35	−5	−45	−105
Total	−59	−48	−922	−210	−1,239	−84	−72	−842	−237	−1,235	−2,474

Source: Elseed A.M. *et al.* (1973) *Archives of Diseases in Childhood*, **48**, 932–936.

8.5.3 Each of 20 animals was given injections of a low and high dose of toxin. After each injection the diameter of the skin lesion was measured (in mm) and these responses are shown below. Ten of the animals (selected at random) had previously been treated with progesterol and the other ten were used as controls. Construct an analysis of variance table to test the significance of the difference between the treatment groups, between doses and the dose × treatment interaction.

Treatment	Progesterol			Control	
Dose of toxin	Low	High		Low	High
Animal			Animal		
1	16·50	20·00	11	16·75	21·00
2	16·00	19·75	12	14·00	20·00
3	15·75	19·00	13	15·50	19·25
4	16·75	20·25	14	14·00	18·50
5	15·50	20·75	15	18·25	22·25
6	15·25	19·25	16	15·00	19·00
7	15·50	18·50	17	14·75	18·75
8	16·50	19·00	18	16·00	19·25
9	17·00	20·50	19	16·75	21·50
10	16·50	20·00	20	16·75	20·00

8.6 MISSING READINGS

8.6.1 A randomized block experiment was planned using five litters of three male mice, one mouse within each litter to each of three diets D_1, D_2 and D_3. However, in the actual experiment only two mice were available in the fourth litter so that one diet, selected at random, was omitted for that litter. Use the growth weights recorded below to test for significant differences between the effects of the three diets.

| | Observed growth weights (gms) | | | | |
| | Litters | | | | |
Diet	1	2	3	4	5
D_1	152	93	110	–	143
D_2	106	77	72	92	127
D_3	109	55	58	59	112

8.6.2 The data below show some of the results, y, of an assessment of techniques for the measurement of systolic blood pressure in infants and children.
  (a) Obtain an estimate of the missing reading, x.
  (b) Calculate the two-way analysis of variance to test for differences between the subjects and techniques ($\Sigma y^2 = 865,829 + x^2$).

| | Technique | | | | |
Subject	Auscultation	Doppler	Flush	Palpation	Total
1	105	110	65	85	365
2	115	115	85	100	415
3	105	105	80	100	390
4	115	115	70	110	410
5	110	116	80	90	396
6	90	95	65	90	340
7	110	110	85	100	405
8	110	110	50	110	380
9	115	110	68	108	401
10	125	125	85	115	450
11	110	110	x	112	$332 + x$
12	120	115	85	110	430
13	120	115	80	105	420
14	105	108	70	100	383
15	100	105	80	85	370
16	85	85	45	75	290
17	130	130	90	120	470
18	105	100	65	105	375
19	105	100	65	105	375
20	110	120	60	100	390
21	86	84	65	90	325
22	110	115	80	110	415
Total	2,386	2,398	$1,518 + x$	2,225	$8,527 + x$

Source: Elseed A.M. *et al.* (1973) *Archives of Disease in Childhood*, **48**, 932–936.

8.7 NON-ORTHOGONAL TWO-WAY TABLES

8.7.1 The following data refer to patients in three diagnostic groups; depression, schizophrenia and alcoholism, who are being treated in a psychiatric hospital. Of interest is the change of social class between the patients' fathers at the time of the patients' birth and the social class of the patients at the time of admission to hospital. The investigator wishes to know whether the change in social class between father and patient varies with diagnosis and/or with the patient's sex. Construct an analysis of variance to test for differences between diagnoses (adjusted for sex) and sex (adjusted for diagnosis).

Distribution of patients by change in social class

Change in social class	Depression Male	Depression Female	Schizophrenia Male	Schizophrenia Female	Alcoholism Male	Alcoholism Female
+2	5	20	0	9	4	3
+1	5	19	6	13	4	4
0	29	57	20	32	15	5
−1	11	29	19	31	7	2
−2	7	6	13	18	5	3
Total, n	57	131	58	103	35	17

8.7.2 In a study of the effectiveness of a programme of oral health education, children from eight schools in the London Borough of Hillingdon were randomly allocated to test or control groups. The test group was examined before and six months after the programme and on each occasion the PM index of gingival inflammation was recorded for each child. The control group was examined at the same times as the test group but did not receive the programme of oral health education. The change in the PM index between the two examinations was determined for each child with the following results:

School	Test group Change in PM index								
	+4	+3	+2	+1	0	−1	−2	−3	−4
DT	2	2	1	4	9	2	2	1	2
BWI	0	2	3	5	8	1	0	2	5
R	2	3	3	4	16	3	0	0	0
SL	1	0	2	4	48	3	1	0	0
M	4	0	2	8	25	0	0	0	0
B	0	0	1	2	10	3	1	0	3
OF	4	1	4	0	9	4	1	1	1
W	1	1	0	5	6	8	3	1	1

School	Control group Change in PM index								
	+4	+3	+2	+1	0	−1	−2	−3	−4
DT	0	0	1	1	6	2	0	0	0
BWI	1	1	2	2	4	0	1	0	0
R	0	0	1	2	5	0	1	0	0
SL	0	1	1	3	17	1	0	0	0
M	2	1	0	4	15	2	0	0	0
B	0	0	0	0	5	3	1	0	0
OF	0	1	1	2	3	0	0	0	1
W	2	0	1	1	5	4	2	0	0

Investigate the significance of the difference between the test and control groups when adjustment is made for schools.

CHAPTER 9

FURTHER ANALYSIS
OF STRAIGHT-LINE DATA

9.1 ANALYSIS OF VARIANCE APPLIED TO REGRESSION

9.1.1 The data of exercise **5.3.1** are the pre-war averages of the net food supply, x, and the infant mortality rates, y, for certain selected countries.

(a) Calculate the linear regression of infant mortality rate on net food supply and test its significance by the analysis of variance.

(b) Verify that the fraction of the total sum of squares explained by the linear regression is the square of the correlation coefficient calculated in exercise **5.3.1**.

9.1.2 The data of exercise **5.3.3** show the consumption of alcohol in litres per year per person aged more than 14 years, x and the death rate per 100,000 population from cirrhosis and alcoholism, y in 15 countries.

(a) Calculate the linear regression of y on x and test its significance by calculating the analysis of variance.

(b) What fraction of the total variability of y is explained by x? How does this relate to the answer to exercise **5.3.3**?

9.3 STRAIGHT LINES THROUGH THE ORIGIN

9.3.1 Fifteen chickens were fed embryonated ova of the nematode *Heterakis galli-narum*. Fifty days later, total daily egg output counts were made on 24 hour faeces collections from each of the birds. The chickens were then killed and the number of female worms in their intestinal tracts (caeca) counted. (See exercise **5.2.2**.)

Chicken number	Number of female *Heterakis*, x	24 hour egg output y
1	2	1,343
2	3	3,067
3	10	15,752
4	24	15,821
5	9	8,762
6	23	19,985
7	12	7,851
8	14	11,704
9	12	13,989
10	1	661
11	4	4,794
12	2	476
13	12	7,067
14	1	346
15	10	8,278

(a) Estimate the slope, b, of the regression line of y on x assuming that the line passes through the origin $(0, 0)$.

(b) Estimate that slope of the line as $b_1 = \Sigma y / \Sigma x$.

(c) Estimate the slope of the line as $b_2 = \Sigma(y/x)/n$.

(d) Assuming the egg count is a Poisson variable, which of these three estimates is preferable?

9.3.2 The data below show the protein absorption at a wavelength of 280 nm for various concentrations of that protein. Calculate the linear regression of absorption on protein concentration so that the regression line passes through the origin.

Absorption	Protein concentration gm/litre
0·08	5
0·19	10
0·22	15
0·30	20
0·38	25
0·45	30
0·51	35
0·60	40
0·71	45
0·78	50

9.4 REGRESSION IN GROUPS

9.4.1 In an assay of heparin a standard preparation is compared with a test preparation by observing the log clotting times (seconds) of blood containing different doses of heparin. Replicate readings are made at each dose level. (See exercise **11.3.2.**)

Log clotting times (y)				Log dose of heparin (x)
Standard		Test		
1·806	1·756	1·799	1·763	0·72
1·851	1·785	1·826	1·832	0·87
1·954	1·929	1·898	1·875	1·02
2·124	1·996	1·973	1·982	1·17
2·262	2·161	2·140	2·100	1·32

Find the regression of log clotting time on log dose for each preparation and test to see if the slopes differ significantly.

9.4.2 Three groups of rats were fed on different diets for the same length of time. Their initial and final weights were recorded in gm. Denote the initial weight of the jth rat in the ith group by x_{ij}, the final weight of the same rat by y_{ij}, and the average initial weight of the n_i rats in the ith group by x_i. Assume that

$$Ey_{ij} = \alpha_i + \beta_i (x_{ij} - x_i)$$

and

$$\text{var } y_{ij} = \sigma^2$$

for $i = 1, 2, 3$ and $j = 1, 2, \ldots, n_i$. Use the data below to show that estimates of β_1, β_2 and β_3 differ significantly.

Group	n_i	$\sum_j x_{ij}$	$\sum_j y_{ij}$	$\sum_j x^2_{ij}$	$\sum_j x_{ij} y_{ij}$	$\sum_j y^2_{ij}$
1	17	1,323	1,233	156,069	146,482	137,657
2	23	2,987	3,596	411,569	495,620	597,588
3	17	2,621	2,691	546,503	558,809	571,793

Source: B.Sc. Pure Science, University of Newcastle-upon-Tyne (1964).

9.5 THE ANALYSIS OF COVARIANCE

9.5.1 During plastic operations to the head, neck or trunk it is inconvenient for the anaesthetist to record the patient's blood pressure from a cuff on the arm. A study was designed to investigate whether blood pressure as measured in the arm could usefully be predicted from a measurement made on the patient's leg. The following data are measurements of systolic blood pressure simultaneously measured in the arm and leg in 36 patients. The anaesthetics used were either halothane or curare. If the linear regression of arm BP, y on leg BP, x were to be used for prediction, would it be necessary to use a separate equation for each anaesthetic or could a single equation be used?

	Halothane				Curare	
Arm BP, y	Leg BP, x	Arm BP, y	Leg BP, x		Arm BP, y	Leg BP, x
115	140	95	95		125	145
100	130	105	130		100	120
115	145	120	140		105	130
130	140	95	110		110	130
95	120	95	115		70	95
100	120	70	100		65	90
130	150	85	110		70	100
110	135	95	115		80	105
125	110	85	110		95	125
90	110	110	110		55	70
95	95				75	100
90	110				50	80
110	130				75	70

9.5.2 The following data are taken from an assay of antihaemophilic globulin by Biggs's method. The table shows the clotting times y (in seconds) for three dilutions of each of five plasmas (A and B being normal subjects, C, D and E being patients). There are two readings at each dilution. The dilutions are equally spaced logarithmically and the working unit x is used instead of log dilution. The table also shows some summary calculations.

Plasma	Dilution	x	y		Summary calculations	
A	1/45	1	16·9	16·9	$\Sigma x = 12$	$\Sigma y = 131\cdot4$
	1/135	2	20·9	21·7	$\Sigma x^2 = 28$	$\Sigma y^2 = 2995\cdot92$
	1/405	3	26·0	29·0	$\Sigma xy = 284\cdot0$	
B	1/45	1	16·3	18·5	$\Sigma x = 12$	$\Sigma y = 127\cdot7$
	1/135	2	20·6	23·0	$\Sigma x^2 = 28$	$\Sigma y^2 = 2776\cdot59$
	1/405	3	24·8	24·5	$\Sigma xy = 269\cdot9$	
C	1/15	0	17·1	18·5	$\Sigma x = 6$	$\Sigma y = 139\cdot1$
	1/45	1	23·8	23·3	$\Sigma x^2 = 10$	$\Sigma y^2 = 3335\cdot75$
	1/135	2	29·0	27·4	$\Sigma xy = 159\cdot9$	
D	1/15	0	18·4	15·4	$\Sigma x = 6$	$\Sigma y = 123\cdot9$
	1/45	1	19·3	20·6	$\Sigma x^2 = 10$	$\Sigma y^2 = 2632\cdot67$
	1/135	2	25·3	24·9	$\Sigma xy = 140\cdot3$	
E	1/15	0	17·3	18·3	$\Sigma x = 6$	$\Sigma y = 129\cdot5$
	1/45	1	22·3	22·2	$\Sigma x^2 = 10$	$\Sigma y^2 = 2844\cdot51$
	1/135	2	24·6	24·8	$\Sigma xy = 143\cdot3$	

(a) Perform a preliminary analysis of variance to confirm the following results.

	Analysis of Variance			
Source	Sum of squares	d.f.	Mean sq.	V.R.
Between subjects	21·17	4	5·29	
Within subjects	(411·52)	(25)		
common slope	375·84	1	375·84	
between slopes	12·09	4	3·02	2·45 $P > 0\cdot05$
deviation of dose				
means from regression	5·09	5	1·02	N.S.
residual (within				
duplicates)	18·50	15	1·23	
Total	432·69	29		

(b) Perform an analysis of covariance to test the differences between the positions of the regression lines for the five plasmas.

(c) Obtain corrected mean values of y corresponding to $x = 1\cdot5$ and their standard errors.

(d) What conclusion can be drawn from (c) regarding the differences between the plasmas?

9.5.3 Refer to exercise **9.4.1**. Analysis of variance showed no significant difference between the slopes of the two regression lines. Perform an analysis of covariance to test the difference in position of the two lines.

CHAPTER 10

MULTIPLE REGRESSION AND MULTIVARIATE ANALYSIS

10.1 MULTIPLE REGRESSION

10.1.1 During the first half of December 1952 the London area experienced periods of fog culminating in one of the most intense on record. The data below show for the first 15 days of that month, the number of deaths occurring in the London Administrative County, the mean atmospheric smoke at County Hall and the mean atmospheric sulphur dioxide content.

Date Dec. 1952	Number of deaths, y	Smoke (mg/m³), x_1	Sulphur dioxide parts/million, x_2
1	112	0·30	0·09
2	140	0·49	0·16
3	143	0·61	0·22
4	120	0·49	0·14
5	196	2·64	0·75
6	294	3·45	0·86
7	513	4·46	1·34
8	518	4·46	1·34
9	430	1·22	0·47
10	274	1·22	0·47
11	255	0·32	0·22
12	236	0·29	0·23
13	256	0·50	0·26
14	222	0·32	0·16
15	213	0·32	0·16

(a) Calculate the linear regression of y on x_1 alone.
(b) Calculate the multiple linear regression of y on x_1 and x_2 and test the significance of inclusion of x_2 in addition to x_1.
(c) Calculate the regression of y on x_2 alone.
(d) Test the significance of the inclusion of x_1 in addition to x_2.

10.1.2 In the study of *Anopheles* larva density two factors involved in the actual collection of larvae are the number of minutes spent dipping, x_1, and the extent of the water surface swept, x_2. The data below were obtained during a malaria survey in Pattukkottai Town and Taluk, Tanjore District, Madras Presidency, India.

Year	Month	Dipping time, minutes, x_1	Area swept, sq. ft, x_2	Larvae collected, y
1937	June	1,187	786	1,728
	July	1,953	1,611	2,758
	August	3,720	3,439	6,309
	September	3,124	3,322	6,776
	October	3,001	3,764	4,487
	November	2,412	2,236	3,801
	December	3,591	4,361	4,303
1938	January	2,585	2,702	2,888
	February	2,933	2,720	3,041
	March	3,878	2,769	5,522
	April	2,829	1,993	5,604
	May	3,120	2,646	5,326
	June	3,823	3,223	8,223
	July	5,505	4,436	15,161
	August	5,350	4,196	13,956
	September	4,572	3,606	12,284
	October	4,825	4,268	10,505
	November	4,393	3,228	8,981
	December	3,479	2,167	5,899
1939	January	2,663	1,438	3,565
	February	1,138	734	2,605
	March	1,242	927	4,671
	April	1,284	1,431	3,486
	May	2,098	1,593	7,519
	June	2,027	1,064	6,777
	July	1,617	1,278	4,120
	August	2,354	1,895	8,153
	September	2,721	1,820	7,086
	October	2,543	1,775	5,041
	November	2,393	1,662	5,384
	December	2,597	1,815	6,484
1940	January	1,936	1,282	4,056
	February	1,139	691	1,931

(a) Calculate the linear regression of y on x_1 alone.
(b) Calculate the linear regression of y on x_2 alone.
(c) Calculate the multiple linear regression of y on x_1 and x_2.
(d) Is the multiple regression of y on x_1 and x_2 a significant improvement on the regression of y on x_1 alone or x_2 alone?

10.3   POLYNOMIAL AND OTHER CURVILINEAR REGRESSION

10.3.1   In a study of the forced oscillation technique for the determination of resistance to breathing in children, 40 children with cystic fibrosis were investigated. The data below show the total respiratory resistance (R_T) in cm H_2O in one second and the height H in cm for each of the 40 children.

Child	R_T	H	Child	R_T	H	Child	R_T	H	Child	R_T	H
1	13·8	89	11	13·5	93	21	7·0	109	31	10·0	138
2	8·2	93	12	11·0	98	22	8·5	118	32	12·7	132
3	9·0	92	13	11·0	103	23	7·4	110	33	6·5	141
4	12·5	101	14	8·8	108	24	7·0	121	34	6·2	136
5	21·1	95	15	9·5	106	25	6·2	120	35	6·0	138
6	6·8	89	16	9·2	109	26	11·6	116	36	7·8	140
7	12·7	102	17	7·0	111	27	5·3	124	37	8·7	140
8	11·0	97	18	6·3	116	28	4·0	123	38	6·2	136
9	8·2	111	19	12·5	116	29	9·8	116	39	4·5	144
10	11·6	103	20	7·9	116	30	9·0	123	40	4·5	145

(a) Draw a scatter diagram to show the association between the dependent variable R_T and the independent variable H.

(b) Calculate the quadratic regression of R_T on height and test the significance of the quadratic term, presenting the results in an analysis of variance table.

$\Sigma R_T = 360·5$, $\Sigma R_T{}^2 = 3666·99$, $\Sigma H R_T = 40,466·7$, $\Sigma H^2 R_T = 4,636,100·3$,
$\Sigma H = 4,618$, $\Sigma H^2 = 544,094$, $\Sigma H^3 = 65,380,876$, $\Sigma H^4 = 8,004,858,434$.

Source: Cogswell J.J. (1973) *Archives of Disease in Childhood*, **48**, 259–266.

10.3.2 An experiment was designed to investigate the time taken by cysts of *Entamoeba Histolytica* to settle in water. Cysts of diameters, x, between 11·5 and 20·2 microns were placed in still water at 10°C and the times, y, taken (in seconds) to settle through 720 microns were measured.

Calculate the quadratic regression of settling time on cyst diameter and test the significance of the quadratic term, presenting the results as an analysis of variance.

Diameter of the cyst (microns), x	Time required for cysts to settle (seconds), y	Diameter of the cyst (microns), x	Time required for cysts to settle (seconds), y
11·5	228·2	15·8	115·2
11·5	206·0	15·8	114·4
13·1	182·0	15·8	112·7
13·1	170·1	15·8	110·9
13·1	152·5	15·8	106·8
14·4	148·9	15·8	106·0
14·4	146·5	15·8	105·9
14·4	144·0	15·8	104·5
14·4	141·7	15·8	103·6
14·4	139·1	17·3	104·0
14·4	136·9	17·3	102·2
14·4	133·8	17·3	100·1
14·4	130·6	17·3	98·1
14·4	128·8	17·3	93·4
14·4	126·5	17·3	92·1
14·4	125·7	17·3	91·3
15·8	125·6	17·3	90·0
15·8	124·9	18·7	88·2
15·8	124·2	18·7	84·0
15·8	120·6	18·7	82·5
15·8	120·5	18·7	76·3
15·8	118·5	18·7	73·0
15·8	117·8	20·2	74·8
15·8	116·0	20·2	66·0

Source: Chang S.L. (1945) *Amer. J. Hyg.*, **41**, 156–163.

10.3.3 Refer to exercises **5.3.1** and **9.1.1**. Inspection of the plot of infant mortality against net food supply suggests that a curve may fit better than a straight line. Fit a quadratic regression to the data and test the significance of the quadratic term.

G

10.4 MULTIPLE REGRESSION IN THE ANALYSIS OF NON-ORTHOGONAL DATA

10.4.1 A randomized blocks experiment was planned using five litters of three male mice, one mouse within each litter to each of three diets D_1, D_2 and D_3. However, in the actual experiment only two mice were available in the fourth litter so that one diet, selected at random was omitted for that litter. The data can be analysed as a randomized blocks experiment (see exercise **8.6.1**) or a similar analysis can be achieved using multiple regression on the dummy variables x_1, $x_2 \ldots x_6$ defined by:

$x_1 = 1$ if an observation is from litter 1 and 0 otherwise
$x_2 = 1$ if an observation is from litter 2 and 0 otherwise
$x_3 = 1$ if an observation is from litter 3 and 0 otherwise
$x_4 = 1$ if an observation is from litter 4 and 0 otherwise
$x_5 = 1$ if an observation is from diet D_1 and 0 otherwise
$x_6 = 1$ if an observation is from diet D_2 and 0 otherwise

Observed growth weights(gm)

Diet	L_1	L_2	L_3	L_4	L_5
			Litters		
D_1	152	93	110	—	143
D_2	106	77	72	92	127
D_3	109	55	58	59	112

Calculate the analysis of variance to test for differences between diets and litters.

10.4.2 In a trial of trishydroxymethyl-amino-methane (THAM) and sodium bicarbonate in the treatment of severe idiopathic respiratory distress syndrome, 25 infants were treated with THAM and 25 with sodium bicarbonate, allocation of infants to treatments being random. In addition, the time of onset of spontaneous respiration (minutes) and birthweight (kg) were recorded for each infant. Define the response variable $y = 0$ if the infant died and $y = 1$ if the infant survived. Let $x_1 = 1$ if the treatment was THAM and $x_1 = 0$ if the treatment was sodium bicarbonate. Let x_2 be the time at onset of spontaneous respiration (in minutes) and x_3 the birthweight in kg. The results were:

For the infants who died

Infant	y	x_1	x_2	x_3	Infant	y	x_1	x_2	x_3
1	0	1	2	1·050	15	0	0	8	1·225
2	0	1	2	1·175	16	0	0	10	1·262
3	0	1	0·5	1·230	17	0	0	0	1·295
4	0	1	4	1·310	18	0	0	2	1·300
5	0	1	0·5	1·500	19	0	0	3	1·550
6	0	1	10	1·600	20	0	0	0	1·820
7	0	1	0·5	1·720	21	0	0	0·5	1·890
8	0	1	0	1·750	22	0	0	5	1·940
9	0	1	6	1·770	23	0	0	10	2·200
10	0	1	2	2·275	24	0	0	0	2·270
11	0	1	0	2·500	25	0	0	0	2·440
12	0	0	7	1·030	26	0	0	2	2·560
13	0	0	0·5	1·100	27	0	0	0	2·730
14	0	0	0	1·185					

and for the infants who survived

Infant	y	x_1	x_2	x_3	Infant	y	x_1	x_2	x_3
28	1	1	0·5	1·130	40	1	1	0	3·640
29	1	1	0	1·575	41	1	1	0	2·830
30	1	1	15	1·680	42	1	0	1	1·410
31	1	1	4	1·760	43	1	0	2	1·715
32	1	1	1	1·930	44	1	0	2	1·720
33	1	1	0	2·015	45	1	0	4	2·040
34	1	1	0	2·090	46	1	0	5	2·200
35	1	1	0	2·600	47	1	0	2	2·400
36	1	1	0	2·700	48	1	0	1	2.550
37	1	1	10	2·950	49	1	0	0·5	2·570
38	1	1	3	3·160	50	1	0	0	3·005
39	1	1	0·5	3·400					

These results yield:

$$\Sigma y = 23, \quad \Sigma y^2 = 23, \quad \Sigma x_1 = 25, \quad \Sigma x_1^2 = 25, \quad \Sigma x_2 = 127 \cdot 0,$$
$$\Sigma x_2^2 = 927 \cdot 00, \quad \Sigma x_3 = 98.747, \quad \Sigma x_3^2 = 216 \cdot 41875,$$
$$\Sigma x_1 y = 14, \quad \Sigma x_2 y = 51 \cdot 5, \quad \Sigma x_3 y = 53 \cdot 071.$$

10.4.2—*contd.*

(a) Calculate the multiple regression of y on x_1, x_2 and x_3.
(b) Test the significance of each regression coefficient.
(c) Test the significance of the multiple regression by the analysis of variance.
(d) Comment on the use of a dummy variable for y in this example.

Source: Van Vliet P.K.J. *et al.* (1973) *Archs. Dis. Childh.* **48**, 249–255.

10.5 LINEAR DISCRIMINANT FUNCTIONS

10.5.1 Refer to exercise **10.4.2**. The multiple regression of y on x_1, x_2, x_3 yields:

$$Y = -0.2970 + 0.1459x_1 + 0.0010x_2 + 0.3450x_3$$

The values of Y predicted by the equation for the 27 infants who died ($y = 0$) and for the 23 infants who survived ($y = 1$) are as follows.

Infants who died

0·2133	0·2563	0·2738	0·3051	0·3669	0·4114	0·4429	0·4527
0·4659	0·6359	0·7114	0·0657	0·0831	0·1119	0·1341	0·1489
0·1498	0·1536	0·2409	0·3309	0·3556	0·3776	0·4725	0·4862
0·5448	0·5883	0·6449					

Infants who survived

0·2393	0·3923	0·4442	0·4603	0·5158	0·5441	0·5700	0·7459
0·7804	0·8772	0·9423	1·0225	1·1047	0·8253	0·1905	0·2968
0·2985	0·4110	0·4673	0·5331	0·5838	0·5902	0·7398	

(a) Use these results to determine a symmetrical rule to use as an end-point for discriminating between the deaths and survivors.

(b) How many infants in this series would be misclassified by this discriminant function?

(c) The sum of squares due to regression is 2·9955 and the sum of squared residuals is 9·4245. Estimate the generalized distance between these two groups.

10.5.2 The following data relate to the same series of 50 infants with idiopathic respiratory distress syndrome as described in exercises **10.4.2** and **10.5.1**.

Infants who died

No.	Apgar score, x_1	Birthweight, x_2	No.	Apgar score, x_1	Birthweight, x_2
1	5	1·050	15	1	1·225
2	4	1·175	16	1	1·262
3	7	1·230	17	7	1·295
4	4	1·310	18	4	1·300
5	8	1·500	19	4	1·550
6	2	1·600	20	10	1·820
7	9	1·720	21	8	1·890
8	8	1·750	22	4	1·940
9	1	1·770	23	2	2·200
10	5	2·275	24	8	2·270
11	9	2·500	25	8	2·440
12	3	1·030	26	6	2·560
13	7	1·100	27	7	2·730
14	8	1·185			

Infants who survived

No.	Apgar score, x_1	Birthweight, x_2	No.	Apgar score, x_1	Birthweight, x_2
28	7	1·130	40	9	3·640
29	3	1·575	41	9	2·830
30	9	1·680	42	8	1·410
31	4	1·760	43	3	1·715
32	1	1·930	44	7	1·720
33	9	2·015	45	5	2·040
34	9	2·090	46	9	2·200
35	7	2·600	47	5	2·400
36	9	2·700	48	6	2·550
37	4	2·950	49	8	2·570
38	1	3·160	50	8	3·005
39	6	3·400			

$\Sigma x_1 = 296$, $\Sigma x_1^2 = 2,108$, $\Sigma x_2 = 98·747$, $\Sigma x_2^2 = 216·414669$,
$\Sigma x_1 x_2 = 605·107$.

(a) Using the method of separation between groups calculate the linear discriminant function of x_1 and x_2.

(b) Calculate the symmetric end-point for the application of the discriminate function.

(c) Calculate the generalized distance between the two groups.

(d) Draw a scatter diagram of the x_1 and x_2 values and draw on it the line of the discriminate function.

10.5.3 Re-calculate the linear discriminant function for the data of exercise **10.5.2** using the method of multiple regression with a dummy variable for the dependent variable y such that $y = 1$ if the infant survived and $y = 0$ if the infant died.

(a) Present the results in the form of an analysis of variance.

(b) Calculate the generalized distance between the group of infants who survived and the group who died.

CHAPTER 11

DATA EDITING

11.3 LOGARITHMIC AND POWER TRANSFORMATIONS

11.3.1 The infant mortality rate and death rate of children aged 1–4 years between 1931 and 1970 for England and Wales are shown below:

Years	IMR per 1,000 live births	Death rate, aged 1–4 years, per 1,000
1931–1935	62	6·56
1936–1940	55	4·70
1941–1945	50	3·50
1946–1950	36	1·77
1951–1955	27	1·14
1956–1960	23	0·91
1961–1965	21	0·86
1966–1970	18	0·76

(a) Draw a diagram to show the decline between 1931 and 1970 in the infant mortality rate and the death rate of children aged 1–4 years on arithmetic graph paper. Which of the two rates has shown the greater absolute decline?

(b) Draw the diagram on semi-logarithmic graph paper. Which of the two rates has shown the greater proportionate decline?

11.3.2   In an assay of heparin a standard preparation is compared with a test preparation by observing the clotting times of blood containing different amounts (dose) of heparin. Replicate readings are made at each dose level.

Clotting times (sec)				Log dose
Standard		Test		of heparin
64	57	58	63	0·72
71	61	67	68	0·87
90	85	79	75	1·02
133	99	94	96	1·17
183	145	138	126	1·32

(a) Draw scatter diagrams of clotting time (y) against log dose of heparin (x) for the standard preparation and the test preparation.

(b) Do the responses appear to change linearly with log dose of heparin?

(c) Does the variance of y appear to change with log dose?

(d) Take logarithms of the clotting times and re-draw the scatter diagrams.

(e) Has the log transformation affected the linearity of clotting time with log dose of heparin?

(f) Has the log transformation affected the apparent change of variance with log dose of heparin?

11.3.3   In an experiment to compare three consoles, the number of errors made by 5 subjects in an experimental period was recorded.

		Console	
Subject	A	B	C
1	7	8	12
2	1	4	8
3	9	7	9
4	3	3	8
5	1	5	4

Make an appropriate transformation of the data and perform a 2-way analysis of variance to test for differences between consoles and differences between subjects.

11.3.4   The data of exercise **8.2.1** show the survival times of animals in a 3×4 factorial experiment, the factors being (a) three poisons and (b) four treatments.

Box and Cox (1964) point out that the reciprocal transformation has natural appeal for the analysis of survival times since it is open to the simple interpretation that it is the rate of dying.

Re-analyse the data using the reciprocal transformation and compare the results with the results from exercise **8.2.1.** In particular comment on the interaction term in the two analyses.

Source: Box G.E.P. & Cox D.R. (1964) *J. R. Statist. Soc. B*, **26**, 211–252.

11.4 TRANSFORMATIONS FOR PROPORTIONS

11.4.1 The following data show the frequency distribution of microfilaria counts in positive people obtained from a 20 cmm stained finger prick blood film.

Microfilaria count, x	$\text{Log}_{10}\, x$	Frequency	Cumulative frequency	Cumulative percentage	Probit
1	0·00	11	11	13·6	3·90
2	0·30	19	30	37·0	4·67
3	0·48	5	35	43·2	4·83
4	0·60	7	42	51·9	5·05
5	0·67	8	50	61·7	5·30
6	0·78	0	50	61·7	5·30
7	0·85	4	54	66·7	5·43
8	0·90	5	59	72·8	5·61
9	0·95	0	59	72·8	5·61
10	1·00	3	62	76·5	5·72
11–20	1·19	3	65	80·2	5·85
21–30	1·41	4	69	85·2	6·04
31–40	1·55	4	73	90·1	6·29
41–50	1·66	2	75	92·6	6·45
51–60	1·74	0	75	92·6	6·45
61–70	1·82	0	75	92·6	6·45
71–80	1·88	0	75	92·6	6·45
81–90	1·93	1	76	93·8	6·54
91–100	1·98	1	77	95·1	6·65
101–200	2·19	2	79	97·5	6·96
201–300	2·41	1	80	98·8	7·26
301–400	2·55	1	81	100·1	—

(a) Draw the curve of the cumulative percentage against microfilaria count on arithmetic graph paper.

(b) Draw the curve of the cumulative percentage against log microfilaria count on arithmetic graph paper.

(c) Draw the curve of the probit of the cumulative percentage against the log microfilaria count on arithmetic graph paper.

(d) Comment.

Source: Southgate B. (1974) *Trans. roy. Soc. trop. Med. & Hyg.*

11.4.2   The table below shows data for 104 medical students who determined their taste threshold to phenylthiourea (PTC). Although thresholds vary widely between individuals they tend to form two distinct groups called 'tasters' and 'non-tasters'. Genetic factors largely determine group membership but thresholds may also be associated with age and sex.

Phenylthiourea taste thresholds in a
sample of 104 medical students

Concentration, mg/l	No. of students	
0·32	0	
0·63	2	
1·27	9	
2·54	16	Tasters
5·08	23	
10·2	12	
20·3	3	
40·6	0	
81·2	3	
162	5	
325	8	Non-tasters
650	10	
1,300	8	
>1,300	5	

(a) Calculate the cumulative relative frequency distributions of tasters and non-tasters.

(b) Draw histograms to illustrate the frequency distributions of thresholds by concentration mg/l.

(c) Take logarithms of the concentrations and plot the cumulative relative frequency distributions against log concentration of PTC.

(d) Transform the cumulative relative frequencies using (i) arcsines, (ii) probits, (iii) logits, and plot the transformed percentages against log concentration of PTC for both tasters and non-tasters.

(e) Comment on the effect of the log transformation of the PTC concentrations and the arcsine, probit and logit transformations of the relative cumulative frequencies.

CHAPTER 12

FURTHER ANALYSIS OF
QUALITATIVE DATA

12.2 COMPONENTS OF χ^2

12.2.1 In a survey, the diets of 175 pregnant Australian women were classed as either *very poor*, *poor*, *fair*, *good* or *excellent*, according to their nutrient and energy content. The incidence of pre-eclamptic toxaemia (classified as a rise in blood pressure with either albuminuria or oedema, and excessive weight gain) was also recorded.

(a) Do the data below support the theory that the occurrence of toxaemia is related to the diet in pregnancy?

(b) Is there a significant trend in the incidence of toxaemia from the 'very poor' to 'good' dietary groups?

Diet in pregnancy	No. with toxaemia	No. without toxaemia	Total
Very poor	8	11	19
Poor	7	26	33
Fair	6	56	62
Good	4	57	61
Total	25	150	175

12.2.2 The following data are some of the results of a survey of dental caries in five towns and also the fluoride content of the public drinking water. Only children aged 12–14 were included in the survey.

(a) Do a significance test to investigate whether the proportion of children caries free differs from area to area. (See exercise **7.4.1**.)

(b) Do the proportions caries free show a significant trend with the fluoride content of the drinking water?

(c) Test the significance of the departure from linearity.

Area Fluoride, p.p.m.	Surrey and Essex 0·15	Slough 0·9	Harwich 2·0	Burnham 3·5	West Mersea 5·8	Total
Children with caries	243	83	60	31	39	456
Children caries free	16	36	32	31	12	127
Total	259	119	92	62	51	583
% caries free	6·2	30·3	34·8	50·0	23·5	21·8

12.2.3 Pregnancies with retarded intra-uterine growth observed in a clinic were classified as to whether threatened miscarriage occurred and whether the placenta was circumvallate (3 degrees, normal, minor and major) at delivery. See exercise **7.4.4**.

	Placenta			
Miscarriage	Normal	Minor	Major	Total
Threatened	10	18	14	42
Not threatened	36	12	8	56
Total	46	30	22	98

The overall $\chi^2_{(2)}$ is 15·82. Calculate the component of χ^2 due to trend, and hence the component due to departure from the linear trend.

12.3 COMBINATION OF 2 × 2 TABLES

12.3.1 A random sample of students listened to recordings of readings by male readers and another sample of students listened to the same readings by female readers. The students were asked to grade the readers as 'not very effective' or 'very effective' with the following results:

Male student listeners

	Readers		
	Males	Females	Total
Not very effective	76	24	100
Very effective	30	15	45
Total	106	39	145

Female student listeners

	Readers		
	Males	Females	Total
Not very effective	19	46	65
Very effective	10	50	60
Total	29	96	125

(a) Calculate χ^2 to test whether male listeners grade one sex of reader better than the other sex of reader.

(b) Calculate χ^2 to test whether female listeners grade one sex of reader better than the other sex of reader.

(c) Use Cochran's method to pool the results of all the students to test whether students of this type show a preference for a particular sex of reader.

Source: Adapted from University of London, M.Sc. Ergonomics, 1975.

12.3.2   The data below show the cardiovascular mortality of patients in a clinical trial of diabetic therapy. Four diagnostic tests were made on the patients. Patients who were positive on the first test only and patients who were positive on all of the other three tests are included here as two separate groups, A and B, respectively. The patients were randomly allocated to a treatment group (Phenformin) or placebo group (insulin).

Test Group	Group A		Group B	
Treatment group	Phenformin	Placebo	Phenformin	Placebo
No. of cardiovascular deaths	8	5	18	7
Total no. of patients	74	82	130	115

(a) Arrange the data for each test group as a 2×2 table and calculate χ^2 to test for difference in cardiovascular mortality between the Phenformin and placebo groups.

(b) Use Cochran's method to pool the results of the two test groups and test the difference in cardiovascular mortality between the Phenformin and placebo groups.

Source: Gray R.H. (1973) *Med. J. Aust.* **1**, 594–596.

12.3.3   In a study of the efficacy of an influenza vaccine at the University of Minnesota, 599 students received the vaccine while the 607 students who acted as controls received normal saline solution. The students were resident in seven dormitories and the numbers vaccinated and the numbers of hospitalized cases of clinical influenza were as follows:

Dormitory	Number of students		Number of cases	
	vaccinated	controls	vaccinated	controls
Sanford Hall	166	172	8	9
Augsburg Seminary	130	134	1	19
Motley School	108	101	4	16
Thatcher Hall	55	54	1	3
Continuation Center	52	49	2	3
Pioneer Hall	18	22	1	1
Private homes	70	75	1	4
Total	599	607	18	55

Use Cochran's method to pool the results from the seven dormitories and test the significance of the difference in influenza incidence between the vaccinated and control groups.

Source: Adapted from Rickard E.R. *et al.* (1945) *Amer. Jour. Hyg.*, **42**, 12–20.

12.5 LINEAR MODELS FOR TRANSFORMED PROPORTIONS

12.5.1 The buffer used in storing semen (for artificial insemination) is thought to have an effect on the number of broken sperms. In an experiment, the semen from four boars was used and stored in four different buffers and 100 sperms from each combination were examined. The following table gives the number of broken sperms in 100 examined.

		Buffer		
Boar	A	B	C	D
1	84	52	26	21
2	58	40	34	11
3	56	27	14	9
4	59	49	30	10

Transform the proportion of broken sperms in each cell of the table using logits. Construct an analysis of variance and test the significance of differences between the buffers, between the boars and the boar $\times$ buffer interaction using the theoretical variance of the logit.

12.5.2 Schistosomiasis is diagnosed in the field by the detection of eggs in the faeces. Three techniques are commonly used which are known as the Bell, Kato and Digestive methods. In cases of heavy infection all of these techniques detect the eggs but in light infections they often fail. Six patients, each with a light infection of schistosomiasis produced faecal samples and each sample was tested ten times by each method. The table below shows the number of times (out of ten) that the tests successfully detected eggs:

		Method	
Patient	Bell	Kato	Digestive
1	1	3	1
2	9	9	9
3	3	3	1
4	9	9	6
5	1	4	3
6	9	9	5

Transform the proportion of correct diagnoses using the logit and test the significance of differences between the methods, the patients and the patient–method interaction using the theoretical variance of the logit.

Source: Teesdale C. Personal communication.

12.5.3 Refer to exercise **12.5.2**. Repeat the suggested analysis using the arc sine transformation and its theoretical variance.

12.6 STANDARDIZATION

12.6.1 The data below relate to maternities in England and Wales in 1960.

Age group of mother	Legitimate			Illegitimate		
	Total mater-nities	Multiple maternities	Per 1,000 total	Total mater-nities	Multiple maternities	Per 1,000 total
Under 20	42,384	274	6·46	9,854	49	4·97
20–24	228,076	2,018	8·85	13,874	124	8·94
25–29	235,879	2,697	11·43	8,414	134	15·93
30–34	146,142	2,093	14·32	5,690	90	15·82
35–39	74,629	1,299	17·41	3,950	81	21·51
40 and over	21,193	273	12·88	1,499	31	20·68
Total	748,303	8,654	11·56	43,281	509	11·76

Examine whether these records provide significant evidence of a difference in the proportions of legitimate and illegitimate maternities which result in multiple births. The sampling errors in the proportions of multiple births among legitimate maternities can be neglected.

12.6.2 The table shows deaths from gall bladder disease and populations at risk by age and two social class groups for males in England and Wales, 1949–1953. Use the indirect method of standardization to compare the mortality experiences of the two social class groups and test the difference in SMR's for significance.

Age (years)	Social class group					
	1 and 2		3, 4 and 5		Total	
	Population, mid-1951 (thousands)	Deaths, 1949–53	Population, mid-1951 (thousands)	Deaths, 1949–53	Population, mid-1951 (thousands)	Deaths, 1949–53
20–24	143	1	1,218	2	1,361	3
25–34	492	7	2,599	7	3,091	14
35–44	660	11	2,603	31	3,263	42
45–54	594	45	2,252	114	2,846	159
55–64	425	133	1,563	252	1,988	385
Total	2,314	197	10,235	406	12,549	603

Source: M.Sc. Medical Statistics, 1973. University of London.

12.6.3 The crude infant mortality rate in 1960 was 32·4 per 1,000 in Alabama and 27·9 per 1,000 in Kentucky. Using the total rates as standards, calculate race adjusted infant mortality rates for the two states and test the significance of the difference between them.

Infant Mortality by Race in Alabama and Kentucky, 1960

	Alabama			Kentucky		
	White	Non-white	Total	White	Non-white	Total
Live births	50,828	30,018	80,846	65,960	6,248	72,208
Infant deaths	1,266	1,350	2,616	1,713	302	2,015
Rate (per 1,000)	24·9	45·0	32·4	26·0	48·3	27·9

12.6.4 Below are shown the number of births and stillbirths in Scotland and Wigtown in particular periods. Calculate the stillbirth rates per thousand live births for the two areas. Standardize the stillbirth rate in Wigtown for the effects of illegitimacy by the use of the data for Scotland and test whether the difference is significant.

	Scotland 1952			Wigtown 1951–53		
	Legitimate	Illegitimate	Total	Legitimate	Illegitimate	Total
Live births	86,116	4,306	90,422	1,611	218	1,829
Stillbirths	2,276	154	2,430	Not available		41

12.6.5 During an epidemic of gastro-enteritis the number of cases and deaths in a city hospital and in all hospitals were as shown below:

Age group (years)	City hospital		All hospitals	
	Cases	Deaths	Cases	Deaths
Under 1	240	48	1,550	341
1–4	140	21	1,880	235
5 and over	20	1	500	16
Total	400	70	3,930	592

(a) Calculate for the city hospital and all hospitals the case mortalities in each age group and for all ages combined.

(b) Find the standardized mortality ratio for the city hospital by the indirect method using the case mortalities by age group of all hospitals as the standard rates.

H

12.6.6   In a study of adult dental health in England and Wales in 1968, the number of males examined, n, and the number found to be edentulous, e, is shown below for each of four regions.

Age	Region The North n	Wales and South West n	Midlands and East Anglia n	London and South East n	All regions n	e	$\%$
16–24	57	25	45	56	183	1	0·55
25–34	74	32	55	92	253	15	5·93
35–44	81	37	69	95	282	46	16·31
45–54	53	23	60	72	208	75	36·06
55–64	76	36	53	87	252	154	61·11
65–74	45	31	24	47	147	114	77·55
75+	13	9	12	23	57	50	87·72
Total examined	399	193	318	472	1,382		
Total edentulous	157	76	96	126	455		
% edentulous	39·3	39·4	30·2	26·7	32·9		

Standardize the crude percentages edentulous in each of the four regions to remove the effect of age from the comparisons, using the overall age specific proportions as standards.

12.7 GOODNESS OF FIT OF FREQUENCY DISTRIBUTIONS

12.7.1 Below is shown the frequency distribution of *Trypanosoma musculi* per oil-immersion field in a thin blood film. If the trypanosomes were randomly distributed throughout the blood film the frequency distribution should follow a Poisson distribution. The Poisson distribution with the same mean density of parasites as the observed distribution is shown.

Number of Trypanosomes per oil-immersion field	Observed distribution	Poisson distribution
0	16	21·22
1	38	32·89
2	30	25·49
3	10	13·17
4	4	5·10
5	1	1·58
6	1	0·40
7+	0	0·15
Total	100	100·00

Test the hypothesis that the trypanosomes are randomly distributed throughout the blood film.

12.7.2 Each of 50 chickens was inoculated with exactly 6 ova of *Heterakis gallinarum*. One month later the chickens were killed and 90 adult worms were recovered from the 300 ova. The distribution of the number of recovered worms per chicken is shown below. If the probability of survival from ova to adult worm were equal for each ova and the same in each chicken, the number of surviving worms per host should follow a binomial distribution with estimated probability of survival $90/300 = 0.30$, as shown. (See exercise **2.5.4.**)

No. of worms per chicken	Observed no. of birds	Binomial distribution $n = 6, \pi = 0.30$
0	9	5·88
1	12	15·13
2	14	16·21
3	11	9·26
4	3	2·98
5	1	0·51
6	0	0·04

Is there evidence against the binomial model of the distribution of worms?

12.7.3   Relatively little is known of the factors which affect the risk of spontaneous abortion in pregnant women. It has been suggested that some pregnant women may be 'abortion prone' while in others the risk may be very small. The data below (see also exercise **2.5.3**) show the number of spontaneous abortions suffered by a sample of 70 women who stated that they wish to have four children and who had been pregnant four times. If the risk of abortion were independent of previous reproductive history and the same for all women, the number of abortions out of four pregnancies should follow a binomial distribution with $n = 4$. The total number of abortions is 81 and hence the estimate of the probability of abortion is $81/(4 \times 70) = 0.2893$. The binomial probabilities of 0, 1, 2, 3, 4 spontaneous abortions are:

Pr (0 abortions) $= 0.7107^4$	$= 0.2551$
Pr (1 abortion) $= 4 \times 0.2893 \times 0.7107^3$	$= 0.4154$
Pr (2 abortions) $= 6 \times 0.2893^2 \times 0.7107^2$	$= 0.2536$
Pr (3 abortions) $= 4 \times 0.2893^3 \times 0.7107$	$= 0.0688$
Pr (4 abortions) $= 0.2893^4$	$= 0.0070$
Total	0.9999

Test the hypothesis that the number of abortions out of four pregnancies is binomially distributed. Comment.

	No. of spontaneous abortions					Total
	0	1	2	3	4	81
Observed no. of women	24	28	7	5	6	70

Source: Doyle P. (1974) M.Sc. Dissertation, L.S.H.T.M.

CHAPTER 13

DISTRIBUTION-FREE METHODS

13.2 ONE-SAMPLE TESTS FOR LOCATION

13.2.1 Two standard procedures for measuring children's height in the field were compared. In the first (A) gentle traction was applied on the mastoid process (resulting in slight lifting) and in the second (B) the child was standing free. Results for twenty children are given below. Carry out a *quick* test to investigate any systematic difference between the two methods.

Child	A	B	Child	A	B
1	108·4	108·2	11	108·8	108·6
2	109·0	109·0	12	110·7	110·0
3	111·0	110·0	13	112·0	112·4
4	110·3	110·5	14	111·6	111·7
5	109·8	108·6	15	109·9	108·9
6	113·1	111·9	16	106·7	106·0
7	115·2	114·8	17	113·5	113·3
8	112·5	112·6	18	110·0	109·9
9	106·3	106·3	19	111·2	110·3
10	109·9	109·7	20	109·7	109·3

13.2.2 A trial was designed to compare the effects of regular apple eating and regular orange eating on dental plaque formation. Thirty children, who all ate the same school dinners were studied for two weeks. During one week each child ate an apple after dinner while in the other week he ate an orange after dinner. The order of apple eating and orange eating was randomized for each child. At the end of each of the two weeks the children were examined and the extent of new plaque formation was measured using Loe's Index which is defined as:

  0 for no plaque,

  1 for plaque which is invisible to the naked eye but which can be detected with
    a probe,

  2 for moderate plaque which is visible,

  3 for heavy deposits of plaque.

Child	Plaque score		Child	Plaque score	
	Apple	Orange		Apple	Orange
1	3	3	16	3	1
2	2	0	17	1	1
3	1	3	18	3	2
4	1	3	19	3	0
5	1	3	20	2	3
6	2	3	21	3	2
7	2	1	22	0	2
8	0	1	23	1	3
9	2	1	24	1	1
10	1	1	25	3	2
11	2	3	26	1	3
12	2	0	27	3	1
13	3	2	28	2	1
14	1	1	29	2	3
15	3	0	30	1	0

Use the sign test to compare the plaque formation after eating the two fruits

13.2.3 The following data show blood glucose levels in mg/kg in rabbits immediately before and two hours after the administration of an analgesic compound. Investigate the effect of analgesia on blood glucose level by applying: (a) the sign test, (b) the Wilcoxon signed rank sum test.

Rabbit number	Before analgesia	After analgesia
1	158	206
2	119	134
3	122	204
4	89	105
5	111	96
6	135	171
7	138	212
8	122	134
9	127	177
10	127	136
11	137	137
12	120	117
13	118	127
14	126	140
15	134	153
16	134	147
17	125	131
18	124	131

13.3 TWO-SAMPLE TESTS FOR LOCATION

13.3.1 Obstetric records of a group of children who died suddenly and unexpectedly, S.U.D., were compared with those of a group of live control children. Observations on the duration of the 2nd stage of labour were as follows:

Time in minutes:

S.U.D.	60, 25, 6, 8, 5, <5, 10, 25, 15, 10
Controls	13, 20, 15, 7, 75, 120*, 10, 100, 9, 25, 30

* Terminated by surgical intervention.

Compare the median duration of labour in the two groups and test the significance of the difference.

13.3.2 In an assay of digitalis, a tincture of digitalis is infused intravenously at a slow constant rate into the heart of an anaesthetized cat until the cat dies. In this experiment 10 cats were treated with a standard tincture and 8 with an unknown tincture. Use a distribution-free test to investigate the difference between the median lethal doses for the two tinctures.

Standard	Unknown
0·378	0·485
0·453	0·655
0·460	0·698
0·494	0·705
0·526	0·708
0·563	0·775
0·570	0·837
0·576	0·946
0·615	
0·723	

13.3.3 The ascorbate excretion (mg per 3 hours) was recorded for 19 students who live and dine in a hall and 13 students who live and dine at home:

Hall: 22, 38, 63, 70, 28, 121, 37, 37, 53, 27, 27, 14, 9, 28, 20, 16, 7, 37, 34
Home: 54, 48, 48, 47, 83, 372, 96, 255, 22, 163, 205, 89, 50

Is there a significant difference between the median ascorbate excretion in the two groups of students?

13.4 RANK CORRELATION

13.4.1 A sample of housewives was shown a list of foods and asked to say whether certain foods had a higher or lower calcium content. From their replies a table was drawn up showing the order in which the whole sample had ranked these foods. The table shows the way in which the over 35 and under 35 age groups ranked foods for their calcium content. Also given is a 'correct' ranking order. How closely does the ranking order given by each age group agree with the 'correct' order?

Foods listed according to their calcium content (highest first)

'Correct' order	Housewives aged under 35 years	Housewives aged over 35 years
Cheese	Milk	Milk
Sardines and pilchards	Cream	Cream
Milk	Cheese	Eggs
Biscuits	Eggs	Cheese
Bread	Sardines and pilchards	Fruit
Cream	Other fish	Liver
Other fish	Liver	Carrots
Green vegetables	Carrots	Sardines and pilchards
Eggs	Green vegetables	Green vegetables
Carrots	Fruit	Other fish
Liver	Other meat	Other meat
Other meat	Bread	Bread
Potatoes	Potatoes	Biscuits
Fruit	Biscuits	Potatoes

13.4.2 Inspection of the plot of the data of exercise **5.3.3** seems to indicate that the data may not be bi-variate normally distributed. Calculate Kendall's rank correlation coefficient τ for this data and test its significance.

CHAPTER 14
SURVIVORSHIP TABLES

14.1 LIFE TABLES

14.1.1 The following life table for Londoners was constructed in 1662 by John Graunt.

Age (years)	Survivors	Age (years)	Survivors
0	100	46	10
6	64	56	6
16	40	66	3
26	25	76	1
36	16	86	0

Use the life table to estimate, for a person on his 26th birthday, (a) the expectation of life, and (b) the probability of survival to age 36, stating any assumptions you make.

Source: M.Sc. Social Medicine, University of London, 1971.

14.1.2 Using the English Life Table, 1950–52, find answers to the following:

(a) What are the probabilities that male and female live births will not survive to their 20th birthday?

(b) What is the probability that a woman aged twenty will survive to the age of fifty?

(c) How does the chance of a man of seventy becoming a centenarian compare with that of a man of sixty?

(d) In what decade of life do most (i) men and (ii) women die?

(e) At what age, of those shown in the table, is the difference between the probabilities of death in the next 10 years of men and women greatest (i) absolutely and (ii) relatively?

(f) The expectations of life of men and women are, respectively,

40·3 and 44·7 years at age 30—difference 4·4 years

14·8 and 18·1 years at age 60—difference 3·3 years

What do these measurements imply regarding the respective mortalities of men and women between age 30 and 60?

English Life Table 1950–52

Age	Males		Females	
x	1_x	$e_x^{\,\circ}$	1_x	$e_x^{\,\circ}$
0	100,000	66·4	100,000	71·5
5	96,186	64·0	97,019	68·7
10	95,866	59·2	96,794	63·9
15	95,601	54·4	96,608	59·0
20	95,151	49·6	96,300	54·2
30	93,820	40·3	95,311	44·7
40	91,968	31·0	93,778	35·3
50	87,591	22·2	90,656	26·3
60	75,823	14·8	83,646	18·1
70	52,350	9·0	67,835	11·0
80	21,130	4·9	36,118	5·8
90	2,184	2·6	6,079	3·1
100	23	1·7	161	2·1

14.1.3 Below are shown age specific death rates, $_nm_x$, of males in England and Wales 1950–52, and the corresponding probabilities of dying in the age group, $_nq_x$. The latter values were calculated by refined actuarial methods for the construction of English Life Table No. 11.

From the specific death rates for Aberdeen City, also given, calculate the survivors at different ages from a thousand births (the l_x column of an abridged life table) on the assumption that for each age group ratios of $_nq_x$ to $_nm_x$ in Aberdeen and England and Wales are the same. The infant mortality rate in Aberdeen in 1950–52 was 30·2 per thousand births.

Death Rates of Males 1950–52

Age group in years	England and Wales $_nm_x$	$_nq_x$	Aberdeen City $_nm_x$
1–4	0·00136	0·00567	0·00131
5–14	0·00061	0·00608	0·00059
15–24	0·00116	0·01142	0·00106
25–34	0·00159	0·01570	0·00143
35–44	0·00288	0·02891	0·00365
45–54	0·00824	0·08116	0·01019
55–64	0·02310	0·20981	0·02690
65–74	0·05519	0·43791	0·06211
75–84	0·12775	0·76472	0·14076

14.2 FOLLOW-UP STUDIES

14.2.1 Below is an extract from a report.

'In the period 1959–63, 199 men in the area were certified to be suffering from pneumoconiosis. They have been followed up for three years to determine mortality. 39 died in the first year after certification, 36 in the second and 26 in the third. Because of movements from the area and deaths from non-associated causes 8, 4 and 16 cases were lost from the follow-up in the first, second and third years respectively.'

Draw up a table to present these data clearly. Calculate the percentage of men who died within 3 years of certification, making allowance for losses from the follow-up.

14.2.2 Soldiers discharged from the army with pulmonary tuberculosis in an African country were followed-up every year to establish what happened to them. Construct a life table to show the number of survivors from an original 1,000 and the numbers dying each year. Assume that those lost to follow-up are an unselected group who are lost evenly throughout the year.

Time	Number found alive	Number died in next year	Number lost in next year
0	506	130	12
1	364	77	28
2	259	50	18
3	191	36	22
4	133		

14.2.3 471 children born in a hospital were traced one year after birth and 5 years after birth to determine mortality. From the data below estimate the percentages of children surviving to one year after birth and five years after birth. Assume that 65% of infant deaths occur in the first six months of life and 70% of deaths during the second to fifth years occur in the first two years of this age interval.

	Known alive at end	Reported dead	No information obtained
First year	330	81	60
Second to fifth years	170	60	100

14.2.4 The following data are some of the results of a study of the persistence of complement-fixing antibodies against Western Equine (W.E.E.) and St Louis (S.L.E.) encephalitis viruses. Patients were followed up for six years after the onset of clinical illness.

Time period since onset (weeks)	W.E.E. patients			S.L.E. patients		
	P	N	L	P	N	L
0–12	323	2	0	80	1	0
13–25	321	7	0	79	6	0
26–38	314	35	32	73	5	8
39–51	247	15	23	60	1	2
52–103	209	43	45	57	5	9
104–155	121	28	52	43	16	2
156–207	41	12	11	25	11	6
208–259	18	5	11	8	2	2
260–311	2	2	0	4	3	1

P is the number of positive patients under observation at the beginning of the time period.

N is the number of patients becoming negative during the time period.

L is the number of patients lost to follow-up during the time period while still positive.

    Present these results in the form of the l_x column of a life table to show the percentage of patients for each illness who remain positive at the start of each time period after making allowance for those lost to follow-up.

Source: Stallones R.A. *et al.* (1964) *Amer. Jour. Hyg.* **79**, 16–28.

CHAPTER 15

SEQUENTIAL METHODS

15.2 SEQUENTIAL ESTIMATION

15.2.1 A doctor wishes to estimate the mean age at diagnosis of patients referred to his clinic for a certain complaint. He would like to obtain the mean value with a precision of ± 2 years, and interprets this as corresponding to a standard error of 1 year.

Below are given the sum and sum of squares of the ages (to last birthday) of successive groups of 10 patients. Approximately how many patients' ages would the doctor need for calculation of the mean?

What estimate would you give of the number of patients required to reduce the standard error to 6 months?

Patients	Σx	Σx^2
1–10	512	27,575
11–20	516	27,326
21–30	566	32,856
31–40	530	28,352
41–50	550	31,103
51–60	553	31,615
61–70	521	27,606
71–80	563	32,293
81–90	524	27,780
91–100	592	35,327
101–110	573	33,633
111–120	547	31,035

15.3 SEQUENTIAL TESTS

Patient number	Treatment	Survival or death	Patient number	Treatment	Survival or death
1a	A	S	30	N	D
1	N	D	35	N	D
2	A	D	37	A	D
3	A	S	36	A	S
5	A	S	39	A	D
6	A	D	45	N	D
8	N	D	3a	A	S
9	N	D	31a	A	S
11	A	S	32a	A	S
12	N	D	51	N	D
13	N	D	40	N	D
14	A	D	42	A	D
15	A	S	43	A	S
16	A	S	47	N	S
17	N	D	48	N	D
18	N	D	49	A	D
19	A	D	52	A	D
20	N	D	41	A	S
21	A	S	46	A	S
26	N	D	50	A	S
28	A	D	53	N	D
25a	N	S	54	N	D
26a	N	S	55	A	D
27a	A	S	56	N	D
28a	A	S	58	A	D
29a	N	D	59	A	D
30a	N	D	60	N	D
10	N	S	62	A	D
7	A	D	63	A	D
22	A	S	64	N	D
23	A	S	65	A	D
25	N	S	57	N	D
27	A	S	61	A	D
34	N	D	66	N	S
29	N	S	67	N	D
32	A	D	68	A	D
31	A	S	69	N	D
33	N	D	33a	N	D
24	N	S	34a	N	D
38	N	S			

15.3.1 The above results were obtained in a trial to compare the proportions of deaths in patients with tetanus receiving either a large dose of tetanus antitoxin given therapeutically (A) or no antitoxin (N). The treatment was allocated randomly and the results are given in the order in which they were received by the statistician.

It was decided during the planning of the trial that if the difference in the probabilities of death were as much as, say, 75% versus 50% then the trial should detect a significant difference. Verify that this difference would give $\theta = 0\cdot75$.

Construct a chart corresponding to the following plan in which $\theta = 0\cdot75$ $2\alpha = \beta = 0\cdot05$.

n	Upper boundary, y
8	8
11	9
15	11
18	12
21	13
23	13
26	14
29	15

(For the lower boundary, y, has negative sign)

Pair the data as you, the statistician, receive them and for each pair determine the preference for A or N if any, and plot the results on your chart. What conclusions can be drawn?

I

CHAPTER 16

STATISTICAL METHODS IN EPIDEMIOLOGY

16.2 RELATIVE RISK

16.2.1 In a retrospective study of the relationship between the use of oral contraceptives and thromboembolic disease, the women were classified according to whether they smoked 0–14 or 15+ cigarettes per day. The results were:

Cigarettes per day	0–14		15+	
	Thromboembolic patients	Controls	Thromboembolic patients	Controls
Oral contraceptives:				
Used	12	8	14	2
Not used	25	84	7	22
Total	37	92	21	24

(a) Calculate the relative risk of thromboembolic disease among users compared with non-users of oral contraceptives for the group who smoke 0–14 cigarettes per day, and test the significance of its logarithm.

(b) Calculate relative risk for women who smoke 15+ cigarettes per day and test the significance of its logarithm.

(c) Do the two log. relative risks, calculated in (a) and (b) differ significantly?

16.2.2   At a large dental hospital 75 patients were admitted for surgery suffering general gingival inflammation and pathological pocketing. Their smoking habits, as reported by the patients are shown below. A control group of patients, not suffering severe periodontal disease, were selected from the wards of the nearest general hospital. They too were asked their smoking habits.

Smoking category	Periodontal patients	Control patients
Non-smokers	10	15
Cigarette smokers	25	28
Pipe smokers	40	32

(a) Calculate the relative risk of severe periodontal disease for cigarette smokers and pipe smokers compared with non-smokers and test the significance of the log relative risks.

(b) Comment on the choice of the controls and indicate how this might affect the interpretation of the results.

16.2.3   In a study of the association between cigarette smoking and lung cancer, 1,357 male lung cancer patients were compared with 1,357 controls in terms of their cigarette consumption as follows:

	Cigarette consumption daily						
	0	1–	5–	15–	25–	50+	Total
Lung cancer patients	7	49	516	445	299	41	1,357
Controls	61	91	615	408	162	20	1,357

Calculate the relative risks of lung cancer in each of the five smoking groups compared with the non-smokers.

16.2.4 A retrospective case-control study was undertaken to examine the association between endometrial carcinoma and the use of oestrogens in post-menopausal women. There were 317 cases of endometrial carcinoma which were individually matched with 317 controls from the same hospital. The matching criteria were age at diagnosis and year of diagnosis. The 317 controls were patients with cervical carcinoma, ovarian cancer or carcinoma of the vulva.

(a) The table below shows the numbers of cases and controls who had previously taken oestrogens for at least six months prior to the diagnosis of carcinoma.

	Cases	Controls
Oestrogen used	152	54
Oestrogen not used	165	263
Total	317	317

Calculate the relative risk of endometrial carcinoma ignoring the matching.

(b) The data below shows the previous use of oestrogen in the 317 matched pairs.

	Controls	
Cases	Oestrogen used	Oestrogen not used
Oestrogen used	39	113
Oestrogen not used	15	150

Use McNemar's test (section **4.7**) to test the association between use of oestrogen and endometrial carcinoma. Recalculate the relative risk allowing for the matching. Source: Smith D. *et al.* (1975) *New Engl. J. Med.* **293**, 1164–1167.

16.3 DIAGNOSTIC TESTS

16.3.1 The table gives the results of a comparison between the indications of the presence of diabetes given by tests of urine and blood in 1,000 subjects. Calculate indices of the sensitivity and specificity of the urine test as an indication of raised blood sugar. What factors may affect these results? How might the validity of the blood test itself be assessed?

		Blood test	
		+	−
Urine test	+	10	30
	−	160	800

Source: M.Sc. Social Medicine, University of London, 1972.

16.3.2 In a method for early diagnosis of lung cancer a score is given for each of a number of clinical signs and the sum of the scores is an index for the patient. It is found that the indices for patients who develop lung cancer have a mean of 0·80 and a standard deviation of 0·10. The corresponding mean and standard deviation for the patients who do not develop the disease are 0·42 and 0·12. Suppose the value 0·6 is taken as a dividing point for early diagnosis and assuming that the distributions of the indices are normal, draw a rough diagram of the two distributions of indices. Mark on your diagram the proportion, A, of the patients with an index greater than 0·6 who do not develop lung cancer and the proportion, B, with an index less than 0·6 who develop lung cancer.

Using a table of the normal distribution estimate the proportion, A, of false positives and the proportion, B, of false negatives, and hence estimate the sensitivity and specificity of the early diagnostic procedure.

16.3.3 An investigation was set up at a hospital to study the accuracy of the diagnosis of salpingitis according to a set of clinical criteria, as it had been noticed that salpingitis was sometimes confused with other conditions (such as appendicitis, ectopic pregnancy, ovarian tumour, etc.). All patients provisionally diagnosed as suffering from salpingitis were subjected to laparascopy so that the diagnosis could be confirmed before treatment started. A count was also kept of patients suffering from the conditions most often confused with salpingitis, so that an estimate could be made of the proportions of wrongly diagnosed patients.

It was found that of 63 patients provisionally diagnosed as suffering from salpingitis, 10 were in fact suffering from other conditions and of 937 patients admitted with provisional diagnosis of appendicitis, ectopic pregnancy, ovarian tumour, etc., 9 were in fact found to have salpingitis.

(a) Estimate the sensitivity, specificity and Youden's index for the provisional diagnosis of salpingitis, in this hospital.

(b) What proportion of the total number of patients had incorrect provisional diagnoses? What is the ratio of correctly diagnosed salpingitis patients to incorrectly diagnosed as suffering from salpingitis?

(c) If the provisional clinical diagnosis were used to estimate the proportion of this hospital population suffering from salpingitis, what would be the result? What is the true proportion?

(d) A group of 62,500 women aged 15–44 was screened for salpingitis using the same set of clinical criteria and 1,625 women were provisionally diagnosed as suffering from salpingitis. If it can be assumed that the sensitivity and specificity of the test in the screening survey is the same as in the hospital patients, what is the provisional estimate of the prevalence of salpingitis in the screened population and what is the best estimate of the true prevalence?

CHAPTER 17

BIOLOGICAL ASSAY

17.1 INTRODUCTION

17.1.1 The data below show the lethal doses in an assay of a sample of digitalin in terms of the international standard digitalis powder. Take logarithms of the doses and estimate the potency of the digitalin sample in units per mg of digitalin giving 95% confidence limits.

Lethal Doses

Digitalin sample (mg per kg)	Standard digitalin (units per kg)	
5·3	1·18	1·33
5·6	1·46	1·43
6·5	1·55	1·74
7·1	1·56	1·40
6·1	1·35	1·85
6·6	1·81	1·59
	1·63	1·78

17.2 PARALLEL LINE ASSAYS

17.2.1 In an assay of the vitamin B content of a yeast preparation, various doses of the standard or test preparations are introduced into a medium in which bacteria (*L. fermenti*) are growing and the response is a measure of the turbidity of the culture. Three measures of turbidity were made at each of three doses of the test and standard preparations, as shown below:

Standard Preparation			
Dose (mμg vit. B$_1$)	3	5	7
Log dose	0·48	0·70	0·85
	332	402	439
Turbidity	347	385	439
	322	394	470
Test Preparation			
Dose (mg yeast)	0·025	0·075	0·150
Nominal dose	1	3	6
Log nominal dose	0	0·48	0·78
	312	423	522
Turbidity	306	451	519
	317	459	515

(a) Calculate the analysis of variance to check the validity of the parallel line model.

(b) Estimate the potency of the test preparation and obtain 95% confidence limits for the true potency.

17.2.2 In an assay of a preparation F against a standard preparation of vitamin D, the response was the degree of bone healing in rats which had developed rickets. The test preparation F and the standard were both administered at three doses and the responses are shown below:

Standard Preparation			
Dose (i.u.)	3·5	7	14
Log dose	0·544	0·845	1·146
	0·00	1·50	2·00
	0·00	2·50	2·50
	1·00	5·00	5·00
	2·75	6·00	4·00
	2·75	4·25	5·00
	1·75	2·75	4·00
	2·75	1·50	2·50
	2·25	3·00	3·50
	2·25		3·00
	2·50		2·00
			3·00
			4·00
			4·00

Preparation F			
Dose (mg)	2·5	5	10
Log dose	0·398	0·699	1·000
	2·75	2·50	3·75
	2·00	2·75	5·25
	1·25	2·25	6·00
	2·00	2·25	5·50
	0·00	3·75	2·25
	0·50		3·50

(a) Calculate the analysis of variance to check the validity of the parallel line model.

(b) Estimate the potency of F and obtain 95% confidence limits for the true potency.

Source: Armitage P. (1971) *Statistical Methods in Medical Research*, Chapter **9**. Blackwell Scientific Publications, Oxford.

17.3 SLOPE-RATIO ASSAYS

17.3.1 In an assay of vitamin B_6 in the dried contents of rumina of calves a test preparation was compared with a standard. The standard preparation contained 0·01 μg pyridoxine per ml. The response, y, is in units of $10^3 \times$ optical density and two measurements are made at each of two doses of the standard and test preparations and in addition two blank or zero doses are made.

Dose (ml)	Blank	Standard	Test
0	95, 95		
½		150, 155	203, 200
1		190, 200	280, 268

Estimate the potency of the test preparation relative to the standard preparation and its standard error.

Source: adapted from Clarke P.M. (1952) *Biometrics*, **8**, 370–377.

17.3.2 In an assay of nicotinic acid in a meat extract, five concentrations of a standard nicotinic acid preparation and three of a solution prepared from the meat extract were inoculated in duplicate tubes with a standard culture of *Lactobacillus arabinosus*. Two blanks were also inoculated. After inoculation each tube was titrated with sodium hydroxide to give a measure of acidity.

μg Nicotinic acid per tube	ml NaOH		ml solution per tube	ml NaOH	
0·05	3·5	3·2	1·0	4·9	4·8
0·10	5·0	4·7	1·5	6·3	6·5
0·15	6·2	6·1	2·0	7·7	7·7
0·20	8·0	7·7			
0·25	9·4	9·5			

Blank tubes 1·5, 1·4 ml NaOH

Estimate the potency of the solution relative to the standard preparation and its standard error.

Source: Data of Kent-Jones D.W. & Meiklejohn M. Cited by Finney D.J. (1947) *J. R. Statist. Soc.* Supplement **9**, 46–91.

17.4 QUANTAL RESPONSE ASSAYS

17.4.1 In an assay of two pertussis vaccines A and B, groups of ten mice were given doses of the vaccines and then challenged by a large dose of living organisms. The doses and the numbers of survivors are shown below:

Dose	Log dose	Survivors from 10 mice	
		Vaccine A	Vaccine B
25	1·4	0	0
100	2·0	4	1
400	2·6	6	2
1,600	3·2	9	6
6,400	3·8	10	10

Estimate the potency ratio of B in terms of A.

17.4.2 A new insecticidal preparation, B, is compared with a standard, A, by spraying groups of 20 flies with varying concentrations in a standard quantity of spray medium. The following numbers killed were observed:

Concentration	A	B
0·8	4	6
1·2	11	14
1·8	16	18
2·7	19	20

Further groups of flies were sprayed with the medium alone and a mortality rate of 10% was observed.

By plotting the response curve against the log concentration, estimate the median lethal concentration for A and B and estimate the potency of B relative to A.

ANSWERS TO EXERCISES

CHAPTER 1

1.2.1

Month	Average number of deaths per day	
	Neonatal	Post-neonatal
January	39·5	34·8
February	39·2	31·1
March	41·0	29·8
April	38·0	23·5
May	36·7	17·8
June	35·9	13·7
July	30·9	13·2
August	30·7	12·3
September	30·2	13·0
October	31·7	14·3
November	32·4	16·4
December	33·4	22·5

1.2.2 ———

1.2.3 ———

1.4.1

Frequency distribution of birth weights,
South-West England, 1965

Weight (lb)	Frequency	Weight (lb)	Frequency	Weight (lb)	Frequency
0–	3	5–	1,182	10–	240
1–	40	6–	4,173	11–	39
2–	82	7–	6,723	12–	2
3–	126	8–	4,305	13–	0
4–	364	9–	1,365	14+	1
				Total	18,645

1.4.2

	Frequency		Percentage	
Haemoglobin %	Before MEP	After MEP	Before MEP	After MEP
30–39	2	1	4·4%	1·7%
40–49	7	2	15·6%	3·3%
50–59	14	7	31·1%	11·7%
60–69	10	17	22·2%	28·3%
70–79	8	18	17·8%	30·0%
80–89	2	8	4·4%	13·3%
90–99	2	6	4·4%	10·0%
100–109	0	1	0	1·7%
Total	45	60	99·9%	100·0%

1.4.3 16·3 years.

1.4.4

Skinfold thickness	Frequency	%	Skinfold thickness	Frequency	%
4–	3	2·5	18–	9	7·4
6–	6	5·0	20–	6	5·0
8–	19	15·7	22–	6	5·0
10–	23	19·0	24–	3	2·5
12–	17	14·0	26–	1	0·8
14–	14	11·6	28–	0	0·0
16–	13	10·7	30–31·9	1	0·8
			Total	121	100·0

1.4.5

Sprayable area (sq ft)	Frequency	Sprayable area (sq ft)	Frequency	Sprayable area (sq ft)	Frequency
160–	2	220–	18	280–	23
170–	3	230–	22	290–	9
180–	6	240–	23	300–	11
190–	10	250–	37	310–	8
200–	14	260–	25	320–	8
210–	16	270–	13	330–339	2

1.4.6

Trypanosomes per cell	Frequency		Percentage	
	Exp. 1	Expt. 2	Expt. 1	Expt. 2
0	10	4	5·2	3·1
1	26	27	13·5	21·1
2	33	27	17·2	21·1
3	30	20	15·6	15·6
4	27	16	14·1	12·5
5	25	17	13·0	13·3
6	16	12	8·3	9·4
7	6	2	3·1	1·6
8	5	1	2·6	0·8
9	5	2	2·6	1·6
10+	9	0	4·7	0·0
Total	192	128	99·9	100·1

1.4.7

	Age (yrs)			Sex		HBsAg status		Total
	0–14	15–29	30+	Male	Female	+ve	−ve	
In hospital	34	82	53	119	50	124	45	169
Not in hospital	85	108	93	167	119	238	48	286
Total	119	190	146	286	169	362	93	455
% In hospital	28·6	43·2	36·3	41·6	29·6	34·3	48·4	37·1

1.5.1

Hospital group	Mean	Median	Mode
A	3·35	3	3
B	5·42	6	6
C	4·84	5	6
D	3·26	1	1

1.5.2

BCG vacc.	Mean	Median	Mode
Oral	5·40	5	3
Intradermal	4·37	4	3
None	3·30	3	3

1.5.3 Mean 6·8, Median 5, Mode 3.

1.5.4

Cohort:	pre 1925	1925–34	1935–44	1945–54
Median age:	16·1	16·6	15·8	15·6

1.6.1. $\bar{x} = 14\cdot10$ mm, $s = 5\cdot03$ mm, 116 observations out of 121 or 95·9% lie within $14\cdot10 \pm 2 \times 5\cdot03$ mm.

1.6.2 BCG oral: $s^2 = 6\cdot86$ mm^2, $s = 2\cdot62$ mm
BCG intradermal: $s^2 = 2\cdot95$ mm^2, $s = 1\cdot72$ mm
No BCG vaccination: $s^2 = 2\cdot14$ mm^2, $s = 1\cdot46$ mm

1.6.3

Group	Median	Interquartile range
Antitoxin:	about 24 yrs	about 16 to 31 yrs
No antitoxin:	about 23 yrs	about 16 to 36 yrs

1.6.4

Measure	Rainfall	Temperature	Relative humidity
Range	6·17 in	1·90°F	13·0%
Mean	3·53 in	72·23°F	78·2%
Std. Dev.	2·30 in	0·64°F	2·8%
C. of V.	65·3%	0·89%	3·6%

CHAPTER 2

2.2.1 (a) 0·09, (b) 0·52, (c) 0·22, (d) 0·056, (e) 0·120, (f) 0·101, (g) 0·326, (h) 0·543.

2.2.2 (a) 0·061, (b) about 9 lb 10½ oz, (c) about 4 lb 9½ oz.

2.2.3 (a) 0·20, (b) 0·04, (c) 0·00672, (d) 0·8926.

2.3.1 (a)

Sequence	Probability	Sequence	Probability
MMMM	0·0693	MFFM	0·0679
MMMF	0·0709	FMFM	0·0643
MMFM	0·0664	FFMM	0·0633
MFMM	0·0675	MFFF	0·0554
FMMM	0·0603	FMFF	0·0582
MMFF	0·0642	FFMF	0·0589
MFMF	0·0628	FFFM	0·0569
FMMF	0·0611	FFFF	0·0527

(b) x: 0   1   2   3   4
    Pr(x):   0·0527   0·2294   0·3835   0·2651   0·0693
(c) $\pi = 0.5172$
    x: 0   1   2   3   4
    Pr(x):   0·0543   0·2328   0·3741   0·2672   0·0716

2.4.1 (a) 2·0689, (b) 0·9778, (c) 0·9988.

2.4.2 mean, 4·5; variance, 8·25.

2.5.1 (a) 0·4219, (b) 0·4219, (c) 0·1406, (d) 0·0156.

2.5.2 0·07776.

2.5.3 (a) 0·2893.

(b) Number of abortions: 0   1   2   3   4
    Expected no. women: 17·86   29·08   17·75   4·82   0·49

(c) No.

(d) Binomial assumptions of constant probability of abortion, independence
    between pregnancies, etc. are invalid.

2.5.4

No. worms per chicken: 0   1   2   3   4   5   6
Binomial Frequency: 9·88   15·13   16·21   9·26   2·98   0·51   0·04

2.6.1 —

2.6.2 0·(...)

2.6.3

No. trypanosomes per field:	0	1	2	3	4+
No. fields:	21·2	32·9	25·5	13·2	7·2

2.6.4 Mean, 9 stillbirths per month, std. dev. approx. 3.

2.6.5 (a) 0·814, (b) 0·168, (c) 0·017, (d) 0·001.

2.7.1 (a) 0·93, (b) 0·16.

2.7.2 Estimated percentage of births premature is 5·5%. From normal approximation,
          6·5% of births are premature.

2.7.3 (a) (i) 0·02275, (ii) 0·01321, (b) (i) 0·4207, (ii) 0·02275, (c) 19·3%.

2.7.4 Observed: (a) 81·0%, (b) 90·5%, (c) 99·0%, (d) 111·5%.
          Normal: (a) 80·0%, (b) 90·3%, (c) 99·9%, (d) 110·2%.

CHAPTER 3

3.2.1   (b) 7·6 microns, (c) 0·16 microns.

3.2.2   (a) 2·782, (b) 3·079, (c) 3·110.

3.2.3   If $n = 25$, $SE(\bar{x}) = 0·6$ oz; If $n = 100$, $SE(\bar{x}) = 0·3$ oz; If $n = 625$, $SE(\bar{x}) = 0·12$ oz.

3.2.4   (a) 179·70 to 323·80 sq ft, (b) 5·2%.

3.3.1   (a) In 95% of lots of 50 mosquitoes, the percentage of susceptibles should be within $25 \pm 1·96 \times 6·12\%$.
(b) 6·12%, (c) 85·07%.

3.3.2   (a) 0·22, (b) (i) 0·057, (ii) 0·059.

3.3.3   (a) 2·83%, (b) 24·65%.

CHAPTER 4

4.2.1   (a) Unlikely, $0·01 < P < 0·05$, (b) 17·26 to 19·74 mg/100 ml

4.2.2   Yes, $P < 0·01$.

4.2.3   No, $P = 0·17$.

4.2.4 $t = 2·65$, $\nu = 11$, $P < 0·05$. Probably species *G. secundum*

4.4.1   Yes, $u = 2·92$, $P < 0·01$.

4.4.2   0·067 to 0·215.

4.4.3   0·09 to 0·31.

4.4.4   4·4% to 10·8%, not significantly different to 6·1%.

4.4.5   6·7% to 21·5%, 4·4% to 23·8%.

4.4.6   0·140 to 0·196, 0·135 to 0·201.

4.4.7   (a) 0·75, (b) 95% confidence limits, 0·61 to 0·89.

4.6.1   (a) Yes, $t = 2·90$, $P < 0·02$, (b) $-4·54$ to $-0·62$.

4.6.2   (a) Drugs unlikely to be equal in effect, $t = 4·06$, $P < 0·01$, (b) 0·70 to 2·46 hours.

4.6.3 (a) $t = -2.07$, $0.05 < P < 0.10$, (b) -0.71 to $+0.03$.

4.6.4 (a) 8·9 gm, 3·39 gm, (b) no, $t = 2.63$, $P < 0.02$.

4.6.5 Yes, $t = -4.37$, $P < 0.001$.

4.6.6 $t = -3.36$, $P < 0.01$.

4.6.7 Yes, $u = 3.04$, $P < 0.01$.

4.6.8 $u = 6.94$, $P < 0.001$, 1·04 to 1·87 years.

4.6.9 Yes, A is probably more abrasive, $t = 2.51$, $P < 0.05$, 0·00013 to 0·00159 gm.

4.6.10 Yes, there is evidence to suggest that group O have the larger diameters on average, $u = 3.92$, $P < 0.001$.

4.6.11 Yes, there is evidence to suggest that treated mice have fewer worms, on average, than untreated mice, $t = 2.40$, $P < 0.05$.

4.6.12 Yes, A is probably better, $u = 4.52$, $P < 0.001$, 0·58 to 1·46 surfaces per child per year.

4.6.13 Yes, $t = 4.47$, $P < 0.001$, 0·72 to 1·90 teeth.

4.6.14 Pooled variance, $s^2 = 20,952.7$, $t = 2.50$, $0.01 < P < 0.05$.

4.6.15 $t = 3.39$, $P < 0.01$, 0·049 to 0·214.

4.6.16 $s^2 = 26,307.28$, $t = 7.38$, $\nu = 21$, $P < 0.001$.

4.7.1 (a) Clearance rates: Chloroquine sulphate, 70·1%, new drug 77·7%, (b) 7·6%, 5·5%, (c) between -3.1% and 18·3% (95% confidence limits), (d) there is no strong evidence to suggest that one drug is better than the other.

4.7.2 (a) $u = 2.4$, $P < 0.05$, (b) 4·4% to 43·6%.

4.7.3 (a) $u = 0.3$ not significant, (b) No. 95% confidence limits for the difference between the proportions of mice developing tumours are -0.178 to 0·250. The confidence interval is very wide and very little can be deduced about the size of the true difference between the tumour rates.

4.7.4 (a) From these results, there is no strong evidence of a difference between the two types of letter in their likelihood to elicit useful replies.
(b) 95% confidence limits for the true difference in response rates are -8.4% to 30·4%. Thus on this evidence, one type of letter could elicit a great deal more useful replies than the other.

K

4.7.5   Yes, the proportion of children using A who withdraw is probably greater than the proportion for D, $u = 2 \cdot 84$, $P < 0 \cdot 01$.

4.7.6 $u = 8 \cdot 66$ without continuity correction or $u = 8 \cdot 57$ with the correction $P < 0 \cdot 0001$.

4.8.1 $\chi^2 = 1 \cdot 94$ or $u = 1 \cdot 39$, $P > 0 \cdot 10$, and $\chi^2_c = 1 \cdot 47$ or $u_c = 1 \cdot 21$, $P > 0 \cdot 10$.

4.8.2 $\chi^2 = 4 \cdot 60$ or $u = 2 \cdot 14$, $P < 0 \cdot 05$, but $\chi^2_c = 3 \cdot 72$ or $u_c = 1 \cdot 93$, $P > 0 \cdot 05$.

4.8.3 $\chi^2 = 4 \cdot 59$ or $u = 2 \cdot 14$, $P < 0 \cdot 05$, but $\chi^2_c = 3 \cdot 70$ or $u_c = 1 \cdot 92$, $P > 0 \cdot 05$.

4.8.4 $P = 0 \cdot 0019$.

4.8.5   (a) $\chi^2 = 11 \cdot 35$, $P < 0 \cdot 001$, (b) $\chi^2 = 7 \cdot 11$, $P < 0 \cdot 01$, (c) $P = 0 \cdot 025$.

4.8.6 $P = 0 \cdot 035$.

4.9.1 $u = 1 \cdot 33$ or $\chi^2 = 1 \cdot 78$, $P > 0 \cdot 10$, $-11 \cdot 0\%$ to $9 \cdot 1\%$.

4.9.2   At 3 feet, $\chi^2 = 1 \cdot 64$, $P > 0 \cdot 10$; at 35 feet, $\chi^2 = 13 \cdot 66$, $P < 0 \cdot 001$.

4.9.3 $\chi^2 = 0 \cdot 00$, NS.

4.10.1   Worker A: (a) Yes, $F = 3 \cdot 16$, $P < 0 \cdot 001$.
                         (b) No, $t = 0 \cdot 7$.
            Worker B: (a) No, $F = 1 \cdot 10$.
                         (b) Yes, $u = 5 \cdot 06$, $P < 0 \cdot 001$.

4.10.2   Yes, the variance appears to be less at 6 a.m., $F = 6 \cdot 13$, $P < 0 \cdot 01$.

4.10.3   No strong evidence against the assumption, $F = 1 \cdot 09$.

CHAPTER 5

5.2.1   (b) $Y = 9 \cdot 24 + 1 \cdot 1137x$.

5.2.2.   (b) $Y = 792 \cdot 9 + 777 \cdot 0x$.

   (c) The regression coefficient, $b = 777 \cdot 0$, is an estimate of the daily egg output per worm.
   (d) Clearly the line should pass through the origin. Reasons for its not passing through the origin include sampling error and the possibility that the assumption of a linear model may be inappropriate. (See e.)
   (e) It is believed that the egg output of certain helminths is depressed if large numbers of worms are present. Thus the assumption of a constant average egg output per worm may be false.

5.2.3 (b) Not through the whole range of parasitaemia levels. At levels less than about 500 the relationship appears to be linear.
(c) $Y = 11\cdot88 + 0\cdot1819x$.

5.3.1 $r = -0\cdot81$. There is no evidence from these data that a plentiful food supply, of itself, causes a reduction in the infant mortality rate. High infant mortality rates are caused by many interrelated biological and social factors with which food supply is associated.

5.3.2 $r = -0\cdot97$. The strong correlation arises because both variables show a definite trend with time. There is no reason to suppose that increasing the number of post-graduate awards will, of itself, cause the death rate to fall.

5.3.3 $r = 0\cdot94$.

5.3.4 $r = 0\cdot63$.

5.3.5 (b) Males $r = 0\cdot34$, Females $r = 0\cdot74$.
(c) All students $r = 0\cdot73$.

5.3.6 (b) $r = -0\cdot65$.
(c) $Y = 1,676 - 3\cdot23x$.

5.4.1 (a) $76\cdot1\%$, $15\cdot5\%$.
(b) $0\cdot1746$.
(c) $t = 0\cdot65$, not significant.

5.4.2 $t = 7\cdot1$, $\nu = 27$, $P < 0\cdot001$.

5.4.3 $t = 9\cdot8$, $\nu = 13$, $P < 0\cdot001$.

5.4.4 (a) $t = 6\cdot57$, $\nu = 59$, $P < 0\cdot001$.
(b) 1,353 per 100,000.
(c) 1,061 to 1,646 per 100,000.
(d) $96\cdot7\%$.

5.4.5 (a) $t = 4\cdot64$, $\nu = 28$, $P < 0\cdot001$.
(b) $t = 4\cdot64$, $\nu = 28$, $P < 0\cdot001$. Identical to test of significance for the slope, b.
(c) When $x = 1\cdot0$, 95% confidence interval is $9\cdot40$ to $11\cdot98$.
When $x = 1\cdot5$, 95% confidence interval is $12\cdot09$ to $14\cdot19$.
When $x = 2\cdot0$, 95% confidence interval is $13\cdot88$ to $17\cdot32$.
(e) $7\cdot50$ to $18\cdot78$.
(f) $r(y-Y, x) = 0$, SD (residuals) $= s = 2\cdot70$.
(g) The residuals are generally negative in the early and late years and positive in the middle period. This indicates that perhaps a second factor which varied in this way would improve prediction or may have caused systematic departures.
(h) $0\cdot62$, 0 to $1\cdot44$.

(i) Inspection of the plot of the data suggests (a) it may not be linear, (b) the variance of MI declines with the spleen rate (this impression can be confirmed by analysis). The residuals also suggest the data are not linear or that some other factor is operating. In general predictions outside the range of the data assume the relation is linear, the variance is constant and no other disturbing variables are present. The calculated confidence limits take no account of departures from assumptions. It would be surprising if the relationship between November spleen rate and malaria index is anything like it was 30 years ago.

CHAPTER 6

6.2.1 (a) 669, 51%.
(b) 89·3, 7·9%.

6.2.2 (a) 386·8 days.
(b) 376·7 days.
(c) Optimal allocation is 161 men and 39 women giving SE(T) = 307·0 days.

6.2.3 Optimal allocation of total sample: age 4–5 years, 17·5%; age 6–7 years, 20·5%; age 8–9 years, 30·0%; age 10–11 years, 32·0%.

6.5.1 (a) 20, (b) Yes, 80.

6.5.2 (a) 1,800, (b) 1,458.

6.5.3 (a) 399, (b) Impossible.

CHAPTER 7

7.1.1 (a) Analysis of variance.

Source	S Sq	df	M Sq	VR
Between strains	81·21	2	40·61	9·67 ($P < 0.001$)
Within strains	117·56	28	4·20	
Total	198·77	30		

(b)

	Strain	9D	11C	DSC1
	Mean	4·00	7·11	7·67
	SE	0·65	0·68	0·59

Clearly 11C and DSC1 are not significantly different, but they each differ significantly from 9D. One can merely say that the data suggest 9D has the shortest mean time to death.

(c) The within group variance seems lower for 9D than for the other two, which is not surprising since the means differ. We could get a separate s^2 for 9D and pool the other two groups.

	9D	11C and DSC1
Within groups SSq	16·00	101·56
d.f.	9	19
s^2	1·78	5·35
SE	0·42	0·77 and 0·67 respectively

This has no important effect on the conclusions.

7.1.2 (a) Analysis of variance.

Source	S Sq	df	M Sq	VR
Between groups	1,455·23	3	485·08	7·87 ($P < 0.001$)
Within groups	68,123·40	1,106	61·59	
Total	69,578·63	1,109		

(b) Group: A   B   C   D
    SE($\bar{x}$):   0·49   0·47   0·47   0·46
(c) $t = 1·15$, not significant. Pooled mean $= 10·19$ with standard error 0·34.
(d) $t = 2·47$, $0·01 < P < 0·05$.
(e) $t = 1·84$, $0·05 < P < 0·10$.

7.1.3 Analysis of variance

Source	S Sq	df	M Sq	VR
Between groups	7·40	3	2·47	9·97 ($P < 0.001$)
Within groups	4·21	17	0·25	
Total	11·61	20		

The group means differ significantly but no use has been made of the number of injections given to the mice in each group. With this information it would be possible to investigate the dose-response relationship between oestrone and the increase in the inter-pubic gap.

7.2.1

Estimates of variance components

	Usual method	New method
Subjects	79·8 (55·3%)	94·9 (72·6%)
Observers	8·2 (5·7%)	2·2 (1·7%)
Residual	56·4 (39·1%)	33·7 (25·8%)

7.2.2　(a) 1·22, (b) 1·02, (c) 0·39,

(d) The increase in sample size from 100 to 1,000 men may involve extra administrative work, investigator's time and time off work for the men, although all these costs should be related more closely to the number of determinations, nr than to the number of men. An attempt should be made to estimate these costs.

7.3.1

Poison	Treatment			
I	A	C	D	B
II	A	C	D	B
III	A	C	D	B

7.3.2

Locality:	Windermere	R. Stour	Grassmere	R. Kennett	Wimbourne	R. Leam	Avon
Mean:	0.559	0·497	0·482	0·473	0·390	0·342	−0·054

7.3.3　A　B　C　D　E　F

7.4.1　$\chi^2_4 = 80\cdot2$, $P < 0\cdot001$. The fluoride content of the drinking water and the percentages of children caries free in the five areas are:

	Essex	Slough	Harwich	Burnham	West Mersea
F. ppm	0·15	0·9	2·0	3·5	5·8
% caries free	6·2	30·3	34·8	50·0	23·5

While it may appear that caries prevalence is associated with the fluoride content of the drinking water this test cannot prove a causal relationship.

7.4.2　$\chi^2_3 = 4\cdot29$, $P > 0\cdot10$.

7.4.3　$\chi^2_3 = 8\cdot98$, $P < 0\cdot05$.

7.4.4　$\chi^2_2 = 15\cdot85$, $P < 0\cdot001$.

7.5.1　$\chi^2_{18} = 28\cdot5$, $0\cdot05 < P < 0\cdot10$.

7.5.2　(a) $\chi^2_{12} = 19\cdot7$, $0\cdot05 < P < 0\cdot10$.
(b) $\chi^2_9 = 14\cdot18$, $P > 0\cdot10$, (c) Yes.

7.5.3　$\chi^2_6 = 31\cdot4$, $P < 0\cdot001$.

7.7.1   Yes, but $\chi^2_9 = 15\cdot6$, $0\cdot05 < P < 0\cdot10$.

7.7.2   No, $\chi^2_5 = 22\cdot9$, $P < 0\cdot001$.

7.7.3   (a) $\chi^2_9 = 1\cdot25$, $P > 0\cdot995$, (b) $\chi^2_9 = 1\cdot71$, $P > 0\cdot995$. The number of accidents appears to be too consistent on both the day and night shifts for them to occur randomly.

CHAPTER 8

8.1.1 ———

8.1.2   (a)

Analysis of variance

Source	S Sq	df	M Sq	VR
Vaccines	0·9217	2	0·4609	13·0 ($P < 0\cdot001$)
Days	3·0070	9	0·3341	9·4 ($P < 0\cdot001$)
Residual	0·6366	18	0·0354	
Total	4·5653	29		

(b) 0·229 to 0·583.

8.1.3

Analysis of variance

Source	S Sq	df	M Sq	VR
Patients	58·1589	4	14·5397	3·77 ($P < 0\cdot05$)
Days	57·7914	6	9·6319	2·50 ($P > 0\cdot05$)
WD × WE	(0·0714)	(1)	(0·0714)	0·02 (NS)
Residual	(57·7200)	(5)	(11·5440)	
Residual	92·4571	24	3·8524	
Total	208·4074	34		

8.2.1

Analysis of variance

Source	S Sq	df	M Sq	VR
Treatments	0·9212	3	0·3071	13·8 ($P < 0\cdot001$)
Poisons	1·0330	2	0·5165	23·3 ($P < 0\cdot001$)
T × P	0·2502	6	0·0417	1·9 ($P > 0\cdot05$)
Residual	0·8007	36	0·0222	
Total	3·0051	47		

8.2.2

Analysis of variance

Source	S Sq	df	M Sq	VR
Operators	592·33	2	296·17	0·57 (NS)
Methods	15·04	1	15·04	0·03 (NS)
O × M	7,264·33	2	3,632·17	6·95 ($P < 0.01$)
Residual	9,403·26	18	522·40	
Total	17,274·96	23		

8.2.3

Analysis of variance

Source	S Sq	df	M Sq	VR
Litters	6·6667	5	1·3333	1·33 ($P > 0.05$)
Treatments	46·7500	3		
Preparations	(16·3333)	(1)	(16·3333)	16·33 ($P < 0.001$)
Doses	(30·0833)	(1)	(30·0833)	30·08 ($P < 0.001$)
P × D	(0·3333)	(1)	(0·3333)	0·33 (NS)
L × T	8·5000	15	0·5667	0·57 (NS)
Residual	24·0000	24	1·0000	
Total	85·9167	47		

8.3.1 (a)

Analysis of variance

Source	S Sq	df	M Sq	VR
Rabbits	475·2525	3	158·4175	6·79 ($P < 0.05$)
Days	435·2425	3	145·0808	6·21 ($P < 0.05$)
Doses	1,190·6025	3	396·8675	17·00 ($P < 0.01$)
Residual	140·0800	6	23·3467	
Total	2,241·1775	15		

(b) SE (any dose mean) = 2·416
dose D_1, $\bar{y} = 11·78$
dose D_2, $\bar{y} = 22·88$
dose D_3, $\bar{y} = 28·95$
dose D_4, $\bar{y} = 35·15$

8.3.2

Analysis of variance

Source	S Sq	df	M Sq	VR
Rows	0·1024	4	0·0256	0·69 NS
Columns	0·2144	4	0·0536	1·45 NS
Concentrations	144·2624	4	36·0656	976·51
Residual	0·4432	12	0·0369	
Total	145·0224	24		

8.4.1

Analysis of variance

Source	S Sq	df	M Sq	VR
Temperatures (unadj.)	6725·8095	6	1120·9682	13·46, $P < 0·005$
Thermometers (adj.)	7665·9048	6	1277·6508	15·34, $P < 0·005$
Residual	666·0952	8	83·2619	
Total	15,057·8095	20		

8.5.1

Analysis of variance

Source	S Sq	df	M Sq	VR (a)	VR (b)
Between men	23·5483				
Smoking	16·0067	1	16·0067		20·58, $P < 0·005$
Pairs	3·6533	5	0·7307		< 1, NS
Residual	3·8883	5	0·7777 (b)	9·00, $P < 0·005$	
Within men	7·1300				
Specimens	3·8400	1	3·8400	44·48, $P < 0·005$	
Spec. ×					
Smoking	2·4267	1	2·4267	28·11, $P < 0·005$	
Residual	0·8633	10	0·0863 (a)		
Total	30·6783	23			

8.5.2 (a)

Analysis of variance

Source	S Sq	df	M Sq	VR (a)	VR (b)
Subjects	5,083·9048	20	254·1952		3·20, $P < 0·01$
Observers	0·0953	1	0·0953		< 1, NS
Error	1,587·4047	20	79·3702 (b)	1·82 $P < 0·05$	
Techniques	43,242·5000	3	14,414·1667	330, $P \ 0·05$	
T × O	198·2381	3	66·0794	1·52 $P > 0·05$	
Error	5,227·2619	120	43·5605 (a)		
Total	55,339·4048	167			

L

(b) Technique means: A: $-3\cdot40$ mmHg; D: $-2\cdot86$ mmHg; F: $-42\cdot00$ mmHg; P: $-10\cdot64$ mmHg. Standard error of any technique mean is $1\cdot02$ mmHg.

8.5.3

Analysis of variance

Source	S Sq	df	M Sq	VR (a)	VR (b)
Between animals	34·2438				
Treatments	0·0250	1	0·0250		< 1 NS
Residual	34·2188	18	1·9010 (b)	6·59 $P < 0\cdot005$	
Within animals	156·2500				
Dose	150·1562	1	150·1562	520·40 $P < 0\cdot005$	
Dose × Treatment	0·9000	1	0·9000	3·12 $P > 0\cdot05$	
Residual	5·1938	18	0·2885 (a)		
Total	190·4938	39			

8.6.1 Estimate of missing value is $110\cdot5$ gm.

Analysis of variance

Source	S Sq	df	M Sq	adj. M Sq	VR
Diets	4,739·4333	2	2,369·7167	1,961·3833	22·76, $P < 0\cdot005$
Litters	7,266·7333	4	1,816·6833	1,777·4833	20·63, $P < 0\cdot005$
Residual	603·0667	7	86·1524		
Total	12,609·2333	13			

8.6.2 (a) $x = 76\cdot97$ mmHg.

(b)

Analysis of variance

Source	S Sq	df	M Sq	adj. M Sq	VR
Techniques	19,585·4255	3	6·528·4752	6,244·6089	147·0, $P < 0\cdot005$
Subjects	8,303·6861	21	395·4136	394·4162	9·29, $P < 0\cdot005$
Residual	2,633·5902	62	42·4773		
Total	30,522·7018	86			

8.7.1

Analysis of variance

Source	S Sq	df	M Sq	VR
Between cells	31·7644	5		
Sex (adj.)	8·4980	1	8·4980	7·02, $P < 0\cdot01$
Diagnosis (unadj.)	23·2319	2		
S × D	0·0345	2	0·0173	< 1, NS

8.7.1—(*contd.*)

Sex (unadj.)	8·2404	1		
Diagnosis (adj.)	23·4895	2	11·7447	9·70, $P < 0·005$
Within cells	478·0161	395	1·2102	
Total	509·7805	400		

8.7.2

Analysis of variance

Source	S Sq	df	M Sq	VR	
Between cells	71·0085	15	4·7339		
Groups (adj.)	1·8633	1	1·8633	< 1,	NS
Schools (unadj.)	49·9289	7			
G × S	19·2163	7	2·7452	1·16	NS
Within cells	812·6554	344	2·3624		
Total	883·6639	359			

CHAPTER 9

9.1.1 (a) $Y = 359·26 - 0·09583\, x$

Analysis of variance

Source	S Sq	df	M Sq	VR
Regression	56,001·9576	1	56,001·9576	50·16 $P < 0·005$
Residual	30,142·1527	27	1,116·3760	
Total	86,144·1103	28		

(b) Fraction of total S Sq explained by regression is 0·6501. From exercise **5.3.1**, $r = 0·8063$, i.e. $r^2 = 0·6501$.

9.1.2 (a) $Y = -5·99 + 1·9779\, x$.

Analysis of variance

Source	S Sq	df	M Sq	VR
Regression	1680·1803	1	1680·1803	96·61 $P < 0·005$
Residual	226·0797	13	17·3907	
Total	1,906·2600	14		

(b) Fraction of total S Sq explained by regression is 0·8814. From exercise **5.3.3**, $r = 0·9388$, i.e. $r^2 = 0·8814$.

9.3.1 (a) 830·79, (b) 862·56, (c) 819·13, (d) answer (b) is preferable.

9.3.2 $Y = 0·01531\ x$.

9.4.1 Standard $Y = 1·2124 + 0·7353\ x$
Test $Y = 1·3568 + 0·5510\ x$
$t = 1·88, \nu = 16, 0·05 < P < 0·10$

9.4.2

Analysis of variance

Source	S Sq	df	M Sq	VR
Common slope	227,015·0361	1	227,015·0361	9,011, $P < 0·005$
Between slopes	1,113·0977	2	556·5488	22·09, $P < 0·005$
Residual	1,284·8483	51	25·1931	
Total	229,412·9821	54		

9·5.1 (a) Halothane $Y = 18·37 + 0·6995\ x$
Curare $Y = -7·80 = 0·8650\ x$
(b) $t = 0·91, \nu = 32$, NS.
(c) Pooled slope 0·7906; $t = 1·96, \nu = 33, P > 0·05$. For the practical purpose of predicting y from x, it would not make much difference whether or not parallel lines were used; the residual variance is about 102 (mmHg)^2 in either case, so that the standard error of a single predicted value of y for $x = \bar{x}$ is about 10 mmHg which is probably too large for the prediction to be useful.

9.5.2 (b)

Analysis of covariance

Source	Corrected S Sq	df	M Sq	VR
Between plasmas	130·39	4	32·598	21·94, $P < 0·005$
Within plasmas	35·67	24	1·486	
Total	166·06	28		

(c) Plasma A, $\bar{y}_c = 19·73$,
Plasma B, $\bar{y}_c = 19·12$,
Plasma C, $\bar{y}_c = 25·35$,
Plasma D, $\bar{y}_c = 22·82$,
Plasma E, $\bar{y}_c = 23·75$.
SE($\bar{y}_c$) = 0·52 for all plasmas.
(d) Grouping $\bar{y}_c$ implies (A, B) < (D, E) < C.

9.5.3

Analysis of covariance

Source	Corrected S Sq	df	M Sq	VR
Between preparations	0·009505	1	0·009505	3·84, $P > 0·05$
Within preparations	0·042095	17	0·002476	
Total	0·051600	18		

CHAPTER 10

10.1.1 (a) $Y = 171·82 + 63·76x_1$

(b) $Y = 89·51 - 220·32x_1 + 1,051·82x_2$. See analysis of variance table below.

(c) $Y = 144·11 + 256·24x_2$.

(d) See analysis of variance table below.

Analysis of variance

Source	S Sq	df	M Sq	VR
Regression on x_1, x_2	205,098	2	102,549	26·6 $P < 0·005$
Regression on x_1 only	136,450	1	136,450	
x_2 in addition to x_1	68,648	1	68,648	24·5 $P < 0·005$
Regression on x_2 only	164,827	1	164,827	
x_1 in addition to x_2	40,271	1	40,271	14·4 $P < 0·005$
Residual	33,654	12	2,804·5	
Total	238,752	14		

10.1.2 (a) $Y = -364·82 + 2·2320x_1$

(b) $Y = 1691·32 + 1·8551x_2$

(c) $Y = -525·76 + 3·4086x_1 - 1·3624x_2$

(d) Yes. The multiple regression of y on x_1 and x_2 is a significant improvement on the regression of y on x_1 alone and y on x_2 alone.

Analysis of variance

Source	S Sq $\times 10^{-6}$	df	M Sq $\times 10^{-6}$	VR
Regression on x_1, x_2	240·521	2	120·261	
Regression on x_1	226·270	1	226·270	
x_2 in addition to x_1	14·251	1	14·251	4·33, $P < 0·05$
Regression on x_2	143·020	1	143·020	
x_1 in addition to x_2	97·501	1	97·501	29·63, $P < 0·005$
Residual	98·731	30	3·291	
Total	339·252	32		

10.3.1 (b) $R_T = 34·34 - 0·3346H + 0·000978H^2$

Analysis of variance

Source	S Sq	df	M Sq	VR
Regression on H, H^2	124·070	2	62·035	7·809
Regression on H	121·458	1	121·458	15·290
H^2 in addition to H	2·612	1	2·612	$0·329\ P > 0·05$
Residual	293·914	37	7·944	
Total	417·984	39		

10.3.2 $Y = 762·31 - 66·0876x + 1·5858x^2$

Analysis of variance

Source	S Sq	df	M Sq	VR
Regression on x, x^2	46,103·6	2	23,051·8	$363·7\ P < 0·005$
Regression on x	42,731·7	1	42,731·7	$674·1\ P < 0·005$
x^2 in addition to x	3,371·9	1	3,371·9	$53·0\ P < 0·005$
Residual	2,852·4	45	63·39	
Total	48,956·0	47		

10.3.3 $Y = 386·66 - 0·1172x + 0·000004x^2$

Analysis of variance

Source	S Sq	df	M Sq	VR
Regression on x and x^2	56,018·4	2		
Regression on x only	56,002·0	1		
x^2 in addition to x	16·4	1	16·4	< 1, NS
Residual	30,125·7	26	1,158·7	
Total	86,144·1	28		

10.4.1

Regression	Residual S Sq	df
y on x_1, x_2, x_3, x_4, x_5, x_6	603·067	7
y on x_1, x_2, x_3, x_4	4,525·83	9
y on x_5, x_6	7,713·00	11

Analysis of variance

Source	S Sq	df	M Sq	VR
Litters	7,109·93	4	1,777·48	20·63 $P < 0.001$
Diets	3,922·76	2	1,961·38	22·77 $P < 0.001$
Residual	603·07	7	86·15	
Total	11,635·76	13		

10.4.2 (a) $Y = -0.2970 + 0.1459x_1 + 0.0010x_2 + 0.3450x_3$

(b) Individual regression coefficients:

variable	coefficient	$t, \nu = 46$	
x_1	0·1459	1·131	NS
x_2	0·0010	0·056	NS
x_3	0·3450	3·441 $P < 0.01$	

(c)

Analysis of variance

Source	S Sq	df	M Sq	VR
Regression on x_1, x_2, x_3	2·9955	3	0·9985	4·87 $P < 0.01$
Residual	9·4245	46	0·2049	
Total	12·4200	49		

(d) In the usual regression model, y is a normally distributed random variable. In this example y is an arbitrary score defining two groups. For further discussion see exercise **10.5.1**.

10.5.1 (a) $z_o = 0.4696$
(b) 16
(c) $\Delta = 1.1083$

10.5.2 (a) $z = x_1 + 46.9680x_2$
(b) $z_o = 99.8675$
(c) $\Delta = 1.0488$

10.5.3 $Y = -0.2758 + 0.007460x_1 + 0.3502x_2$

Analysis of variance

Source	S Sq	df	M Sq	VR
Regression	2·7514	2	1·3757	6·69 $P < 0.005$
Residual	9·6686	47	0·2057	
Total	12·4200	49		

(b) $\Delta = 1.0487$

CHAPTER 11

11.3.1 (a) Infant mortality rate; (b) death rate aged 1–4 years.

11.3.2 (b) No.
   (c) Yes. The variance appears to increase with log dose.
   (e) The log transform has improved the linearity.
   (f) The variance appears to be less dependent on log dose.

11.3.3 If the errors occur randomly in time, the number of errors made in a given time period should be a Poisson variable, in which case the square root transformation is appropriate.

Analysis of variance

Source	S Sq	df	M Sq	VR	
Subjects	3·8164	4	0·9541	3·816	$P < 0.005$
Consoles	2·2623	2	1·1312	4·525	$P < 0.025$
Residual	1·5294	8	0·1912	0·765	NS
Poisson			0·25		
Total	7·6082	14			

11.3.4

Analysis of variance

Source	S Sq	df	M Sq	VR	
Treatments	20·4147	3	6·8049	28·34	$P < 0.005$
Poisons	34·8774	2	17·4387	72·63	$P < 0.005$
Interaction	1·5702	6	0·2617	1·09	NS
Residual	8·6445	36	0·2401		
Total	65·5068	47			

In the analysis of the transformed data the treatment and poison effects are more significant and the interaction is less significant. Thus an additive model without interaction appears to fit transformed data better than the same model on the untransformed data.

11.4.1 ———

11.4.2

Conc, mg/l	log conc.	Frequency	Relative frequency	Cumulative rel. freq.	$\sin^{-1}\sqrt{p}$	Probit	Logit
0·32	−0·50	0	0	0	0		
0·63	−0·20	2	3·1	3·1	10·1	3·13	−3·44
1·27	0·10	9	13·8	16·9	24·3	4·04	−1·59

11.4.2—(*contd.*)

2·54	0·40	16	24·6	41·5	40·1	4·79	−0·34
5·08	0·71	23	35·4	76·9	61·3	5·74	1·20
10·2	1·01	12	18·5	95·4	77·6	6·68	3·03
20·3	1·31	3	4·6	100·0	90·0		
Total tasters		65	100·0				
81·2	1·91	3	7·7	7·7	16·1	3·57	−2·48
162	2·21	5	12·8	20·5	26·9	4·18	−1·36
325	2·51	8	20·5	41·0	39·8	4·77	−0·36
650	2·81	10	25·6	66·6	54·7	5·43	0·70
1,300	3·11	8	20·5	87·1	69·0	6·13	1·91
>1,300		5	12·8	99·9	90·0		
Total non-tasters		39	99·9				

(e) The log concentrations are easier to plot and because the concentrations double between each entry in the table, the log concentrations are evenly spaced. The cumulative relative frequency curve is approximately sigmoid when plotted against log concentration and nearly linear if the cumulative relative frequency is transformed using arcsines, probits or logits.

CHAPTER 12

12.2.1 Overall $\chi^2_3 = 17\cdot35 \; P < 0\cdot001$
Linearity $\chi^2_1 = 14\cdot88 \; P < 0\cdot001$
Departure $\chi^2_2 = \;\; 2\cdot47$ NS

12.2.2 Overall $\chi^2_4 = 80\cdot22 \; P < 0\cdot001$
Linearity $\chi^2_1 = 45\cdot87 \; P < 0\cdot001$
Departure $\chi^2_3 = 34\cdot35 \; P < 0\cdot001$

12.2.3 Overall $\chi^2_2 = 15\cdot86 \; P < 0\cdot001$
Linearity $\chi^2_1 = 13\cdot41 \; P < 0\cdot001$
Departure $\chi^2_1 = \;\; 2\cdot44$ NS

12.3.1 (a) $\chi^2_1 = 0\cdot94$ with continuity correction, NS.
(b) $\chi^2_1 = 2\cdot10$ with continuity correction, NS.
(c) $\chi^2_1 = 3\cdot98$, $P < 0\cdot05$, preference for female readers.

12.3.2 (a) Group A, $\chi^2_1 = 0\cdot60$, NS
Group B, $\chi^2_1 = 3\cdot21$, $0\cdot05 < P < 0\cdot10$
(b) $u = 2\cdot24$ or $\chi^2_1 = \;\; 5\cdot04$, $P < 0\cdot025$

12.3.3 $u = 4\cdot47$ or $\chi^2_1 = 19\cdot99$, $P < 0\cdot001$

12.5.1

Analysis of variance

Source	S Sq	df	M Sq	VR
Boars	2·2596	3	0·7532	17·4 $P < 0.001$
Buffers	14·9313	3	4·9771	114·7 $P < 0.001$
Interaction	1·1973	9	0·1330	3·1 $P < 0.01$
Theoretical			0·0434	
Total	18·3882	15		

12.5.2

Analysis of variance

Source	S Sq	df	M Sq	VR
Methods	4·2565	2	2·1282	5·31 $P < 0.005$
Patients	46·3645	5	9·2729	23·14 $P < 0.005$
Interaction	5·2763	10	0·5276	1·32 NS
Residual			0·4008	
Total	55·8973	17		

12.5.3

Analysis of variance

Source	S Sq	df	M Sq	VR
Methods	592·0	2	296·0	3·61 $P < 0.05$
Patients	7,292·5	5	1,458·5	17·77 $P < 0.005$
Interaction	722·0	10	72·2	0·88 NS
Residual			82·1	
Total	8,606·5	17		

12.6.1 $u = 2.67$ or $\chi^2 = 7.14$ $P < 0.01$.

12.6.2   Social class groups 1 and 2, SMR $= 1.56$.
Social class groups 3, 4 and 5, SMR $= 0.85$.
$u = 5.94$ $P < 0.001$.

12.6.3   Race adjusted infant mortality rates:
Alabama   29·71 per 1,000 livebirths.
Kentucky   30·99 per 1,000 livebirths.
$u = 1.42$ NS.

12.6.4   Standardized stillbirth rate for Wigtown, 21·87 per 1,000 livebirths. $u = 1.46$ NS.

12.6.5   (a) Case mortality rates, %.

Age	City hospital	All hospitals
under 1	20·0	22·0
1–4	15·0	12·5
5 and over	5·0	3·2
Total	17·5	15·1

12.6.6   Standardized percentages edentulous:
North, 39·83%.
Wales and South West, 35·59%.
Midlands and East Anglia, 32·27%.
London and South East, 26·42%.

12.7.1 $\chi^2_3 = 3\cdot85$ NS.

12.7.2 $\chi^2_3 = 2\cdot99$ NS.

12.7.3 $\chi^2_2 = 14\cdot76$ $P < 0\cdot001$.

CHAPTER 13

13.2.1   Sign test, $u = 2\cdot12$ or $\chi^2_1 = 4\cdot50$ both with continuity correction, $P < 0\cdot05$.

13.2.2 $u = 0\cdot4$, $\chi^2 = 0\cdot16$, both with continuity correction, NS.

13.2.3   (a) $u = 2\cdot91$ or $\chi^2 = 8\cdot47$, both with continuity correction, $P < 0\cdot01$.
(b) $u = 3\cdot10$, $P < 0\cdot01$.

13.3.1   Median duration of labour: SUD group 10 minutes, control group 20 minutes.
$u = 1\cdot65$, $0\cdot05 < P < 0\cdot10$.

13.3.2 $u = 2\cdot58$, $P = 0\cdot01$.

13.3.3 $u = 3\cdot38$, $P < 0\cdot001$.

13.4.1   Age under 35 years, $\tau = 0\cdot34$.
Age over 35 years, $\tau = 0\cdot12$.

13.4.2 $\tau = 0\cdot56$, $u = 2\cdot92$, $P < 0\cdot01$.

CHAPTER 14

14.1.1   (a) 19·4 years, (b) 0·64.

14.1.2 (a) Males 0·04849, Females 0·03700.
(b) 0·94139.
(c) Age 60, 0·00030; Age 70, 0·00044.
(d) 70 to 80 years of age for both sexes.
(e) Absolutely at age 70 years, relatively at age 50 years.
(f) Nothing without further information of life table measures, particularly the numbers surviving.

14.1.3

Age, x	l_x
0	100,000
1	96,980
5	96,450
15	95,883
25	94,882
35	93,543
45	90,115
55	81,070
65	61,263
75	31,071
85	4,891

14.2.1

x	l_x	d_x	p_x	q_x
0	1,000	200	0·80	0·20
1	800	192	0·76	0·24
2	608	152	0·75	0·25
3	456			

54·4% died within 3 years of certification.

14.2.2

Time, x	l_x	d_x
0	1,000	260
1	740	163
2	577	115
3	462	93
4	369	

14.2.3 82·0% survive 1 year.
65·6% survive 5 years.

14.2.4

Time since onset, x	WEE patients l_x	SLE patients l_x
0	1,000	1,000
13	994	987
26	972	913
39	858	846
52	803	832
104	618	753
156	436	466
208	289	233
260	173	166

CHAPTER 15

15.2.1 $n = 81$ patients to reduce the standard error to 1 year.
$n = 324$ patients to reduce the standard error to 6 months.

15.3.1   Boundary crossed at $n = 18$, $y = 12$. There is evidence to suggest that tetanus antitoxin reduces the fatality rate.

CHAPTER 16

16.2.1   (a) Relative risk $=$ 5·04, $u = 3·17$, $P < 0·01$.
(b) Relative risk $= 22·00$, i $= 3·55$, $P < 0·001$.
(c) $u = 1·46$, NS.

16.2.2   (a) Cigarette smokers, relative risk $= 1·34$, $u = 0·59$, NS.
Pipe smokers, relative risk $= 1·88$, $u = 1·34$, NS.
(b) The control group consists of patients from a general hospital who are not suffering severe periodontal disease. Since smoking may affect the chance of a person entering a general hospital, these estimates of relative risk are probably lower than the estimates which would have been obtained from a random sample of persons not suffering severe periodontal disease.

16.2.3

Cigarette consumption	0	1–	5–	15–	25–	50+
Relative risk	1·00	4·69	7·31	9·50	16·08	17·86

16.2.4   (a) Relative risk $= 4·49$.
(b) $u = 8·57$ with continuity correction, $P < 0·001$. Relative risk allowing for matching $= 7·53$.

16.3.1   Sensitivity $= 0·06$, specificity $= 0·96$.

16.3.2   A $= 0·07$, B $= 0·02$, sensitivity $= 0·98$, specificity $= 0·93$.

16.3.3 (a) sensitivity = 0·86, specificity = 0·99, Youden's index = 0·84.
  (b) 1·9%, 5·3.
  (c) 6·3%, 6·2%.
  (d) 2·6%, 1·8%.

CHAPTER 17

17.1.1 Potency estimate 0·25 units per mg.
  95% confidence limits 0·22 to 0·28 units per mg.

17.2.1 (a)

Analysis of variance

Source	S Sq	df	M Sq	VR
Between doses	90,854·4	5		
Preparations	4,802·0	1	4,802·0	30·3 $P < 0.005$
Common slope	85,528·0	1	85,528·0	539·6 $P < 0.005$
Between slopes	317·6	1	317·6	2·0 NS
Non linearity	206·8	2	103·4	< 1 NS
Within doses	1,902·0	12	158·5	
Total	92,756·4	17		

  (b) 95 mμg vitamin B_1 per mg yeast.
    85·1 to 106·1 mμg vitamin B_1 per mg yeast.

17.2.2 (a)

Analysis of variance

Source	S Sq	df	M Sq	VR
Between doses	43·3944	5		
Preparations	0·0118	1	0·0118	< 1 NS
Common slope	36·5893	1	36·5893	26·06 $P < 0.005$
Between slopes	3·7545	1	3·7545	2·67 NS
Non linearity	3·0388	2	1·5194	1·08 NS
Within doses	58·9689	42	1·4040	
Total	102·3633	47		

  (b) 1·46 i.u. per mg.
    0·90 to 2·38 i.u. per mg.

17.3.1 1·88, 0·14.

17.3.2 0·10, 0·0015.

17.4.1 About 0·17.
17.4.2 Median lethal concentration for A is about 1·2 and for B about 1·0. Potency
  of B to A is 1·2.